How to Grow Your Investigative Site

Barry Miskin, M.D., with Ann Neuer

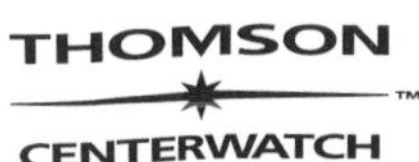

22 Thomson Place · Boston, MA 02210
Tel (617) 856-5900 · Fax (617) 856-5901 · www.centerwatch.com

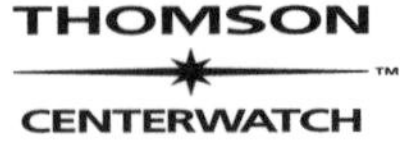

How To Grow Your Investigative Site
by Barry Miskin, M.D., with Ann Neuer

Managing Editor
Sara Gambrill

Publisher
Ken Getz

Design
Liz Abbate

Printed in the United States.
1 2 3 4 5 05 04 03 02

For more information, contact CenterWatch, 22 Thomson Place, Boston, MA 02210. Or you can visit our internet site at http://www.centerwatch.com.

ISBN 1-930624-27-1

Instructions for Obtaining Continuing Medical Education Credit

This book has been planned and produced in accordance with the Essentials and Standards of the Accreditation Council for Continuing Medical Education (ACCME).

With the purchase of the book, the owner is eligible to take an exam and receive four hours of Category 1 credit. The exam and instruction are available through the following web site:

www.centerwatch.com/bookstore/pubs_profs_invguide.html

CONTENTS

INTRODUCTION

For the last couple of years, Ken Getz and I have been talking about writing a book designed to help investigators grow their clinical trials business. Ken and I both felt that as the market for investigative site services matures, there will be a growing need for information aimed at helping the experienced investigator grow his or her research practice to the next level. This guide was created to meet that need.

How to Grow Your Investigative Site provides step-by-step direction for growing a small site into a larger research center. It identifies the subjective and objective criteria signaling you that it is time to expand, and it details the infrastructure and financial controls needed to support this growth. You will find information on budgeting, contracting, patient recruitment, regulatory issues, technology, office systems, keeping your study coordinator, the status of the clinical trials marketplace and more. While some of the information provided is technical and data-driven, there are many personal anecdotes that offer solutions to common problems. We've organized the chapters into two primary categories: practical insights into building infrastructure and into establishing operating controls and processes.

Recognizing that the investigator is not alone in conducting clinical trials, I geared this book toward all the clinical staff participating in the study conduct at the investigative site. For the site-level coordinator, the text offers pointers and templates such as a sample evaluation form to determine study feasibility, universal worksheets and boilerplate contracts. The book provides project managers with tools for patient recruitment and improved standard operating procedures (SOPs). For sponsors, CROs, SMOs and monitors, the book offers insight into the complexities of running a large site and the components needed to optimize performance.

The book represents twenty-five years of personal experience combined with thousands of hours of interviews with industry experts, including sponsors, CROs, SMOs, independent consultants, monitors, quality assurance people, regulatory personnel, coordinators, project managers, auditors, investigators and site administrators. By promising anonymity to those who requested it, I was able to glean some wonderful pearls of information that would not have been available otherwise. As many of you know, the clinical trials industry is small and, at times, secretive.

When I started Palm Beach Research Center (PBRC) in 1993, I had one research center, two coordinators, one small smoking-cessation study and one large dream. Two years later, when annual gross revenues exceeded $200,000 and PBRC was conducting more than ten studies, we expanded the first location from 1200 square feet to 2000 square feet. Subsequently, we've expanded to more than 5000 square feet. This expansion was long overdue. During construction, some of our coordinators were using their laps as desks, and one of our investigators was assigned a shelf as his desk. We had to take turns using the computer.

Shortly thereafter, we were able to justify adding a second site when we secured study contracts for multiple sites and were consistently meeting patient enrollment targets. In 1998, we added our third, fourth and fifth sites in quick succession to accommodate our growing business. We also centralized regulatory, quality assurance and marketing functions at that time.

Today, Palm Beach Research Center is a dedicated research site with five affiliated sites running more than fifty trials. I was only able to achieve this success with the help of some excellent people.

I wish the information in this book had been available when I first started on the path of expanding my research center. It would have saved me much time, thousands of dollars and possibly spared me from learning the hard way—through making mistakes. I only hope that my experiences and the information provided in this book equip the reader with the tools to easily, yet carefully, facilitate growth of his or her clinical trials business. If so, I have accomplished my goal.

Barry Miskin, M.D.
West Palm Beach, Florida

CHAPTER 1

When It's Time to Grow Your Site

- Objective Criteria That Inform the Decision to Grow
- What Is the Status of the Current Marketplace?
- Are You Willing to Either Pay for an Experienced Study Coordinator or Pay for the Training of a New One?
- Should You Start Your Expansion by Focusing on Phase III Trials?
- In Review

If you walk into your site and your files are lining the hallway, or a monitor is waiting for you and two others are on their way, or you find a stack of messages from a few weeks ago that you still haven't answered, you need to think about growing your site. There are other, subtler signs that it is time to grow as well. Growing a site offers the promise of more revenue, but also means paying for additional staff, space and infrastructure with no guarantee of securing enough studies to cover these costs.

With so many variables, it is hard to know if growing is the right choice. You may think that you can continue site operations without making plans to grow. As the number of studies increases, you may assume your current staff can shoulder the additional workload without the benefit of additional hires or additional infrastructure. This approach is shortsighted and will lead to staff burnout, too much paperwork, too little space and difficulties scheduling sufficient time for clinical research while maintaining a traditional medical practice.

Unlike more mature industries with established benchmarks for growth, the clinical trials industry is young and basically lacking in this sort of standardization. There are no standard guidelines suggesting the proper number of study coordinators to hire or the number of square feet needed to optimize operations. But even without specific benchmarks, the investigator will eventually discover that he or she and existing staff can handle only a certain number of studies before reaching capacity. This can happen when gross revenues reach between $200,000 and $350,000. There is no set point, but the number of studies is likely to range between four and six, depending upon their design, duration, frequency of patient visits, number and types of procedures and complexity.

If you plan to maintain your medical practice at its current level, the maximum number of studies you can handle in a capable fashion may be even more restricted without the benefit of expansion. This is due to the fact that clinical studies are loaded with details and activities that make substantial time demands on the investigator. Besides patient visits and the associated procedures and paperwork, there will be more monitoring visits as the number of studies increases. In some instances, you may need to be available to meet with the monitor for several hours.

Signs of an Overloaded Site
The principal investigator is unable to fulfill obligations as an investigator because he or she has too many studies.
Case report forms are not being filled out in a timely fashion.
Regulatory documents are not being submitted in a timely fashion.
Serious adverse events (SAEs) are not being addressed in a timely fashion.
Coordinator and other study staff quit because they are overwhelmed or because they have concerns about good clinical practices not being adhered to.
Telephone calls are not being returned in a timely fashion.
Staff is not happy when a new patient is enrolled in a study protocol.
Coordinator is so busy that he or she cannot sit still for a monitor's visit.

Table 1 Source: CenterWatch interviews

In clinical research, like medicine, there are signs and symptoms that you have reached a point where growth is necessary. Your gut feeling that you could be successful handling more than the one or two studies you are now conducting is a subjective criterion. So is the belief that the in-house patient database will enable you to fill a greater number of appropriate trials. Running out of space to store trial documents, nowhere for the monitors to sit, spending more time at investigator meetings and less time overseeing trial details and on the medical practice are objective criteria pointing toward the need to grow the site.

Example 1 – Not enough space to store documents

Consider the episode of the case report forms (CRFs) stacked in the hallway. I recently attended a conference at a large, well-known university. At one point during the conference, I noticed an interesting phenomenon as I walked through the offices of the Department of Medicine. There were large numbers of binders stacked waist high, lining the walls outside the conference room and around the sides of the walls between offices. On closer inspection, I noted that these were CRFs. Not only is this a major breach of confidentiality and poor space management, but it is also a telltale sign of the need to expand the physical site.

I brought this situation to the attention of the Department Chairman. He was taken aback. He had not realized the gravity of the situation in spite of his passing these stacks daily. The university has since enlarged the size of its clinical research site.

Example 2 – More than one monitor visiting on the same day

A well-known investigator in the Midwest faced the problem of having three monitors arrive on the same day. Two had deadlines and no other alternative, and the third was scheduled. Resourceful as he was, the investigator seated one in the regular monitor room, one in his private bathroom and the third in his RV, which he had had the foresight to drive that day. This doctor knew it was time to grow. With his connections in the mobile home industry, he was able to solve the space problem on a short-term basis by parking his new doublewide trailer outside his office. This worked well until another physician reported him for a zoning violation. He has since moved to a larger office and his business is doing quite well.

Example 3 – The investigator is busier and busier

Studies often start up quickly and with short notice during certain times of the year, particularly in October, November and December. This may present a problem for the investigator who must be available to attend investigator meetings. At that time of year, it is not unusual for the investigator of a growing site to travel every weekend for one or two months in a row to attend startup investigator meetings, end-of-study meetings and mid-study recruitment sessions. In addition, as the investigator starts devoting more time to clinical trials, he or she will have less time to see patients in the medical practice. At this point, the investigator needs to make some serious decisions about recruiting additional investigators. This is an important consideration as the research coordinators must have access to an experienced investigator on weekends in case of an emergency.

Nursing, managerial and office staff are also affected by the increased burden created by the expansion of clinical trials. One example is the office manager who may no longer be able to oversee details of the clinical trials while managing the medical practice. Another is the medical assistant who is so busy taking vital signs and completing paperwork on prospective study patients that the practice patients are kept waiting longer and longer, and eventually walk out (Table 1). These are the costs associated with choosing not to grow when all objective criteria suggest that expanding may be well advised. In deciding not to grow, an investigator may overwhelm him- or herself and the staff with work while limiting the revenues he or she can generate through the conduct of only a few trials at any given time.

Objective Criteria
Do you understand the clinical trials marketplace?
What is the competition in your geographic area?
Should your site remain single specialty or branch out to become multi-specialty?
Are you willing to pay for an experienced study coordinator or invest in the training of a new one?
Do you understand what is involved in accepting studies of various phases or is it best to start building the site with phase III studies?
Are you willing to invest in the infrastructure needed to make this venture a success?
Are you willing to continue learning about Good Clinical Practice (GCP)?
Are you willing to delegate?
Do you want to manage the additional staff required to handle an increased workflow?

Table 2

Source: CenterWatch interviews

Objective Criteria That Inform the Decision to Grow

If any of these scenarios sounds familiar, your site may either be bursting at the seams or becoming noticeably busier. To make an informed decision about growth, it is important to consider a number of objective criteria (Table 2).

Each criterion informs the decision to grow. Also, the criteria are interrelated. For example, the degree to which you invest in infrastructure may depend on the current status of the clinical trials marketplace. The types of specialties you add to your site are a function of the competition in your locale and your relationships with other nearby investigators. Your ability to attract experienced coordinators is also a function of area-wide competition.

The issue of developing infrastructure is very broad and makes up much of the content of this book. Infrastructure will be discussed in the following four chapters. It includes space planning, personnel requirements and business development.

What Is the Status of the Current Marketplace?

If you are considering the expansion of your site, you have probably been successful in conducting a limited number of clinical trials. Translating that achievement into continuing success requires an understanding of the marketplace you are planning to enter.

The clinical trials industry is healthy and growing. The Pharmaceutical Research and Manufacturing Association (PhRMA), which represents the country's leading pharmaceutical and biotechnology companies, reports

Clinical Grant Spending in 2000

Grant Sources	2000 (Projected) in $billions
PhRMA	$2.70
Non-PhRMA	$0.67
Medical Devices	$0.40
NIH	$0.75
TOTAL	**$4.52**

Table 3 Source: CenterWatch

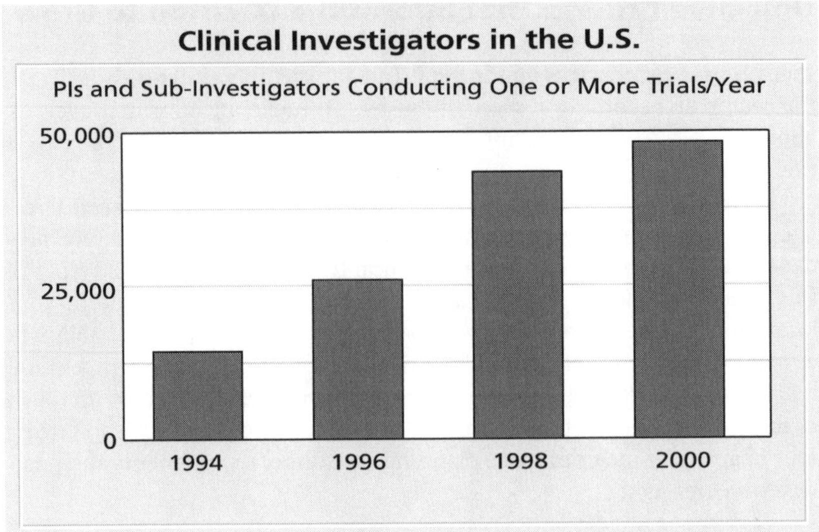

Figure 1 Source: CenterWatch Analysis, FDA

that in 2000, its members spent $22.48 billion domestically on Research and Development for human-use and veterinary-use pharmaceuticals,[i] an 11.8% increase over the 1999 figure.* Of this total, it is estimated that PhRMA members granted $2.7 billion to investigators in 2000 for the conduct of industry-sponsored human clinical trials. It is further estimated that an additional $1.82 billion in investigator grants were funded by the National Institutes of Health (NIH), non-PhRMA sources, and the medical device industry (Table 3). This combined figure of $4.52 billion is a 40% increase over the 1998 level of grant spending (Figure 1).[ii]

There are several factors driving this impressive growth. First, PhRMA members have been increasing their overall R&D budgets every year (Figure 2).[iii] They have also raised the percentage of R&D dollars allocated to the conduct of clinical trials. In 1990, PhRMA members spent $6.8 billion on domestic R&D, and directed 29% of those dollars to phases I through IV clinical trials. By 2001, that percentage rose to approximately 34%. Nearly $24 billion will be spent on R&D in 2001.

As grant sources have been on the rise, so too have the number and size of grants. Sponsors are increasing grant size as a result of having to recruit larger numbers of patients for more complex trials. A survey of forty-five independent for-profit sites conducted by CenterWatch in 2000 revealed that the average grant size of respondents is $56,106, nearly 8% above the 1998 level (Figure 3).[iv] PhRMA reports that its members are growing spending on clinical grants by 16% annually.[v] Dedicated sites also projected that they expected to conduct twenty-nine studies in 2000 as compared to twenty-

* CenterWatch estimates that a substantial majority of these dollars are spent on human-use pharmaceuticals. (CenterWatch, November 2000.)

two studies in 1998. They forecasted 11% to 15% net operating profit margins on revenues of $1.63 million. Nearly 90% of respondents reported that they are profitable.

All is not rosy, however. Although workload and grant size are up, profitability is harder to achieve. When adjusted for inflation, fees received per

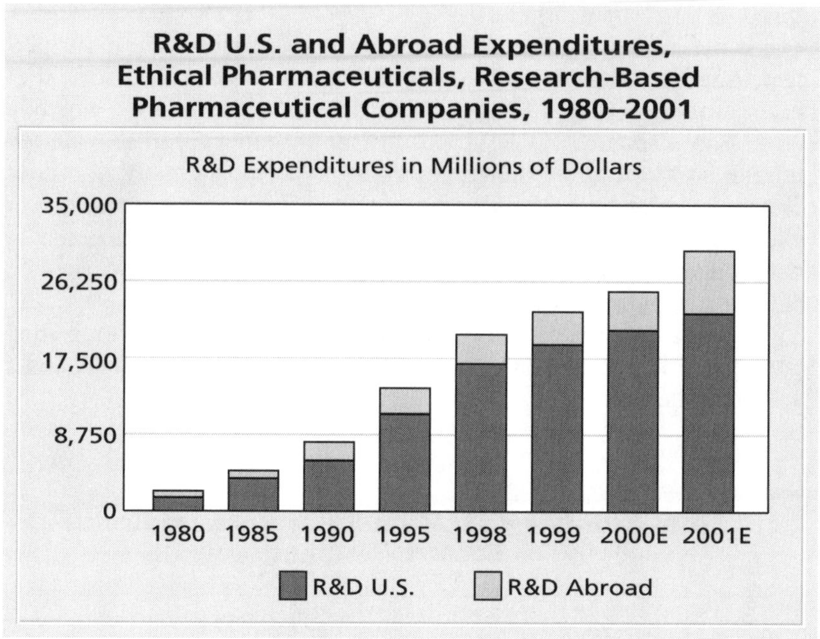

Figure 2 Source: PhRMA Annual Survey, 2001

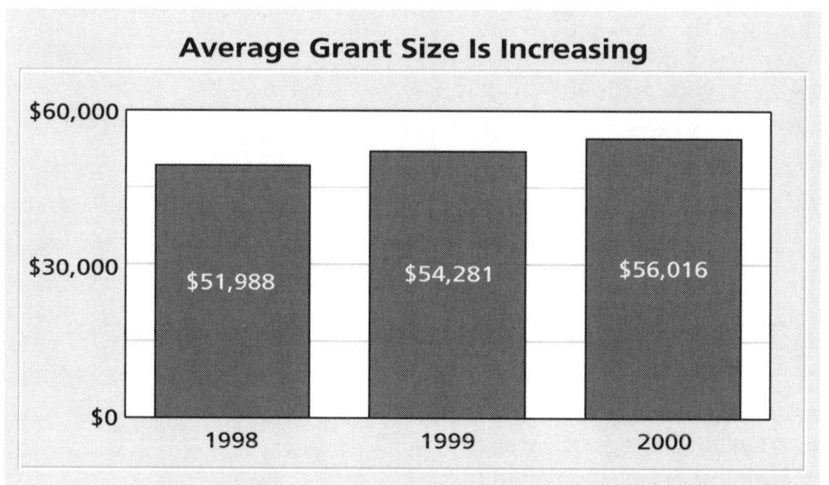

Figure 3 Source: CenterWatch

study subject were essentially flat between 1990 and 2000 mostly because overhead costs rose and protocols required sites to perform 8% to 10% more procedures annually.[vi] In the CenterWatch study, sites reported this increase in the number of required procedures, as well as a noticeable boost in competition for patients and studies due to a flood of new investigators, coupled with longer waits for payment from sponsors or contract research organizations (CROs) in some instances.

Because of the sharp rise in the number of investigators now participating in clinical trials, it is logical to assume that at least some of the less experienced investigators may not be able to determine that a proposed study budget from a sponsor of CRO is insufficient to conduct profitably. Newer, hungrier investigators are sometimes willing to accept any study, regardless of ability to conduct it properly or profitably. This has led to situations in which experienced sites that confront sponsors about the realities of inadequate budgets for particular studies are told that a number of other sites are willing to accept the study budget as is.[vii]

There was a 15% rise in the number of investigators completing Statement of Investigator FDA Form 1572s between 1998 and 2000, and a 226% jump between 1994 and 2000 (Table 4).[viii]

Total Number of Statement of Investigator FDA Form 1572 Filings

Year	Number of 1572s
2000	34,393
1999	28,413
1998	20,331
1990	8,156

Table 4 Source: FDA, DataEdge

As competition becomes stiffer among part-time investigators, there is additional rivalry from the other three venues where clinical studies are conducted. These include:

- Academic Medical Centers (AMCs)
- Dedicated Sites
- Site Management Organizations (SMOs)

As seen in Figure 4, these three categories compose 62% of the industry-sponsored clinical trials market share. Competition for studies and patients is heating up as these study venues align with one or more site networks and study brokers, which are companies dedicated to linking sponsors with experienced investigators.

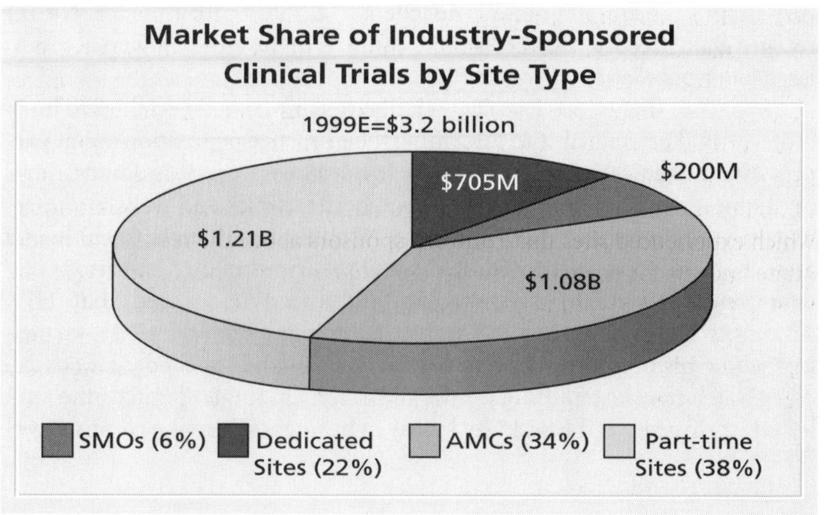

Figure 4 Source: CenterWatch

Although more dollars are currently flowing into investigative sites, it is important to mention that market conditions can and do change. For example, a number of publicly traded contract research organizations were high flyers through much of the late 1990s, yet their stock values declined substantially by 2000 as overhead costs escalated and sponsors cancelled contracts. Cancellation of studies was generally linked to uncertainties experienced by some sponsors in the midst of mergers. By 2001, the downward trend started reversing direction because the abnormal level of study cancellations had abated as mergers were completed, and investors began to view companies in the healthcare sector as a defensive play in an uncertain market.

Prior to adding the second PBRC site, I carefully reviewed market conditions in our geographic area of South Florida. To the best of my ability, I identified all competitive sites and spoke to as many people as possible in my geographic area who worked in this industry and were willing to talk about the type, size and number of ongoing studies. Gathering this information anecdotally seemed to be the only way to gauge the size of the competition because objective criteria, such as number of trials and associated revenues for specific sites, are not publicly available.

As part of my assessment of the competition, I explored the prospects for patient recruitment. Could our area of therapeutic expertise enable us to offer unique services to the 1 million people in our metropolitan area? How could we appeal to the special populations in our area—people over age 65 and people belonging to various ethnic groups—in a way that our competition could not? I thought about the need to staff our site with professionals able to conduct studies that were compatible with our demographics, including drug studies for treatment of signs and symptoms of arthritis, Alzheimer's disease, migraine headache and urinary incontinence. Next, I realized that I needed to approach my contacts in the area who had access to large older populations.

As part of that effort, I spoke with doctors in various specialties to learn if they would be amenable to informing their practice population about participating in clinical trials. I also spoke to administrators of hospitals, nursing homes, rehabilitation centers, public health clinics and walk-in centers to gauge their interest in participation. The public health department in our area and state helped by providing demographic information of various disease states and their prevalence in our area. We learned that HIV, Alzheimer's disease and diabetes were predominant. I interviewed investigators with a history of conducting successful trials and solicited their advice.

While it may be tempting for the site to remain single specialty, the reality is that diversity is the best way to stay in business. There is a comfort level

Company-Financed R&D by Top Product Classes, Ethical Pharmaceuticals, Research-Based Pharmaceutical Companies

Product Class	Estimated 2001 $billions
Cancers, endocrine system, metabolic diseases	$7.4
Central nervous system and sense organ diseases	$7.3
Infective and parasitic diseases	$4.1
Cardiovascular diseases	$3.9
Digestive or genito-urinary system diseases	$1.4
Respiratory system diseases	$1.3
Dermatologic diseases	$0.3

Table 5 Source: PhRMA Annual Survey 2001

attached to conducting trials in your area of expertise, but when making a decision about growth, you will need to offset the cost of additional overhead by accepting studies in many therapeutic areas, instead of just one. Furthermore, studies in all therapeutic areas tend to be cyclical, so by accepting diverse types of studies, you may be able to soften the impact of down cycles in your specific therapeutic area. As the site expands, it should seek to have a steady stream of studies in various phases of startup, in progress and being closed out. The best way to accomplish this is to diversify. As seen in Table 5, the biggest research dollars are spread among various specialties.

There do not appear to be specific benchmarks guiding the decision to go multi-specialty. Anecdotal evidence that I have accumulated over twenty years suggests that principal investigators looking to diversify may try to co-venture with family practitioners or internal medicine specialists to gain access to migraine, hypertension, diabetes, rhinitis and other types of large, broad-based trials. Without this cadre of specialists, you will lose many opportunities to participate in some of the more lucrative clinical trials.

Example 1 – Attracting Central Nervous System (CNS) Studies

Once our young site became successful at handling multiple studies, monitors began to notice. In some instances, we were able to make their jobs easier because during one visit, they could monitor more than one of their studies. As the good news spread, we started receiving offers for more studies in diverse therapeutic areas, including central nervous system (CNS), one of the largest areas of clinical research. First, we obtained a stroke study followed by several migraine trials. Initially, we contracted with primary care physicians, but when we started pursuing more complex CNS studies, we discovered that sponsors required board-certified neurologists for those protocols.

Because PBRC did not have agreements or relationships with board-certified neurologists at that time, the site lost out on several lucrative studies. That was our incentive to seek out these specialists and encourage them to participate in these studies as investigators.

Finding motivated medical specialists with an interest in clinical trials and whose first priority is quality is a special challenge for the owner of a growing site. Once specialists are identified, you will need to assess their knowledge of clinical trials conduct. You may also have to provide some sort of additional training. Although the dangers of "training your competition" and revealing your leads to them are very real concerns, this is a risk that must be taken. Failure to take this risk seriously hinders your potential for expansion.

We have been able to limit the training of the competition by using two techniques. First, we have identified retired specialists who are well known and well respected in our geographic area. This approach has proven to be very successful as these individuals generally are not seeking to build a clinical trials business. Instead, they are seeking an outlet for their talents and energies. Often, they have a broad patient base. Another category is specialists who are disabled from their specialty but are able to work in other therapeutic areas without jeopardizing their benefits.

Are You Willing to Either Pay for an Experienced Study Coordinator or Pay for the Training of a New One?

The study coordinator is key to the ongoing success of a clinical trials operation (see "Hiring and Retaining Your Study Coordinators"). The study coordinator is responsible, in a hands-on fashion, for the running of a research trial, including its many clinical, regulatory and business components. Generally, the best coordinators are detail-oriented, driven, Type A personalities and are registered nurses, licensed practical nurses or medical assistants.

Because of the importance of this position, an investigator should weigh the pros and cons of hiring an experienced versus an inexperienced coordinator who needs to be trained. There are pros and cons to both approaches.

An experienced study coordinator understands the importance of properly completing paperwork, including the case report form. Coordinators who supply perfect or near-perfect reports not only reduce the amount of time the monitor needs to review files, they can also attract business as the word spreads that a particular site consistently maintains excellent records, generating minimal queries. An experienced coordinator, however, can be expensive.

Inexperienced coordinators can be an option as well. Although they are less expensive to hire, they must be trained to be effective, which takes time. Whether they are trainable is unknown upon hire. Monitors visiting the site do not want to train novice coordinators, and may not want to return to a site with an untrained coordinator.

Requiring study coordinators, new and experienced, to become certified by the Association of Clinical Research Professionals (ACRP) or the Society of Clinical Research Associates (SoCRA) shows a commitment to quality and a willingness to invest in the professional development of clinical staff. To sit for the ACRP certification examination, a coordinator must have accumulated a minimum of two years full-time, or four years part-time, clinical trials experience and, at a minimum, be able to enroll study subjects, conduct study subject visits and maintain source documents. Visit www.acrpnet.org for further information. To sit for the SoCRA certification examination, a coordinator must have been employed in the area of clinical research full-time during two of the last five years or in a part-time capacity for 3,500 hours over the past five years; or hold an Associate's or Bachelor's degree in clinical research; or hold an Associate's or Bachelor's degree in science, health science, pharmacy or a related field, and completed 12 undergraduate or graduate credit hours in clinical research. Visit *www.socra.org* for more information.

Should You Start Your Expansion by Focusing on Phase III Trials?

According to the Pharmaceutical Research and Manufacturing Association (PhRMA), $2.83 billion or 42% of the more than $6 billion dollars spent on clinical development in 1999 went to phase III development[ix] (Figure 4). Of that figure, it has been estimated that slightly more than 35% of clinical development dollars are spent on investigative sites.[x] Using that percentage, nearly $1 billion of the $2.83 billion spent on phase III by PhRMA members would go to investigative sites ($2.83 billion x .35).

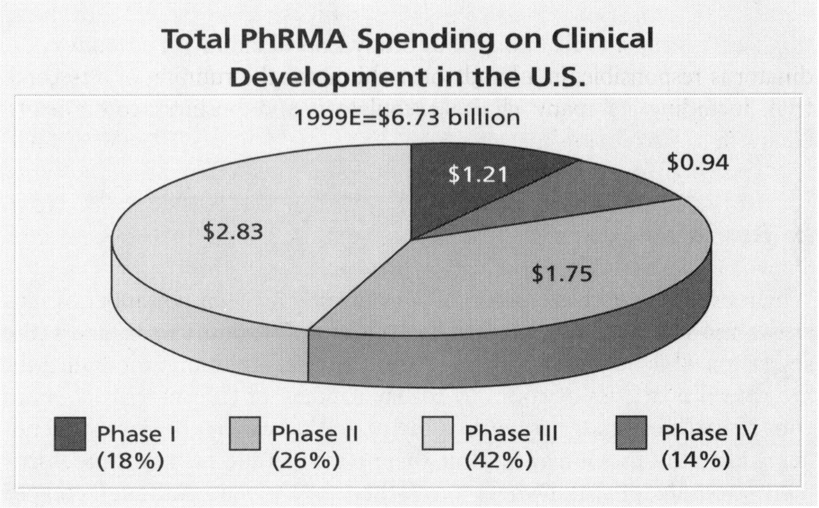

Figure 5 Source: PhRMA

As phase III clinical trials represent a large opportunity, it may be sensible to start out by pursuing this piece of the pie, not only because of the dollars associated but also because some phase III protocols may be less complex than those from other phases (Table 6). Success with a phase III trial will work toward building a site's track record of success. By comparison, a young site that accepts a study that is too complicated, too labor intensive or too difficult to enroll can defeat its own purpose.

Phase I trials may require access to an inpatient facility. Phase II trials may entail multiple and frequent blood draws that have to be precisely timed. To comply with the protocol, patients must remain at the site for long periods of time, so they need to be occupied with some degree of entertainment, food and pleasant surroundings. For these reasons, starting with phase III may be a good strategy.

Some Simpler Phase III Protocols
Limited blood tests
Limited visits
Simple inclusion/exclusion criteria
Universal appeal such as smoking cessation or weight loss

Table 6

In Review

When considering the expansion of your investigative site, a number of subjective and objective criteria must be evaluated. The desire to expand is the key factor. This may stem as much from personal ambition as it does from the objective realities of your day-to-day conduct of clinical trials. Perhaps your research business has reached the point that case report forms are not being filled out in a timely fashion, there is no place to file any more documents, monitors have nowhere to sit when they visit, or staff is starting to quit as they become too overwhelmed.

These objective criteria are parts of the bigger picture, which will ultimately help you realize that the site is too crowded or too bogged down with work, staff is overly stressed and the site cannot accept more studies without adding infrastructure. If you have decided that yes, it's time to address these issues, then it's also time to move ahead with expansion.

If this is the case, it may be time to grow your site. When making this critical decision, identifying the required steps will enhance your chances for success. Taking the time to learn the market, study the competition, explore the possibility of moving from a single specialty site to a multi-specialty site, consider more phase III studies and invest in real infrastructure are some of the tough issues you will need to address.

You will need to address changes and growth in the following areas before and during the growth of your site:

- Space Planning
- Personnel Requirements
- Computerization and Enhancement of Office Systems
- Budgeting

- Partnerships
- Regulatory Issues
- Patient Recruitment and Protection
- Training
- Development of Standard Operating Procedures

References

i *www.phrma.org/publications*, accessed January 23, 2001.

ii "Grant Market to Exceed $4 Billion in 2000," *CenterWatch*, Vol. 7, Issue 11, November 2000, p. 1.

iii *www.phrma.org/publications*, accessed January 26, 2001.

iv "Uphill Growth for Dedicated Sites," *CenterWatch*, Vol. 7, Issue 12, December 2000, p. 7.

v "Grant Market to Exceed $4 Billion in 2000," *CenterWatch*, Vol. 7, Issue 11, November 2000, p. 7.

vi Op. cit. *CenterWatch*, p. 6.

vii "Uphill Growth for Dedicated Sites," *CenterWatch*, Vol. 7, Issue 12, December 2000, p. 7.

viii DataEdge, Ft. Washington, Pa. January 29, 2001.

ix "Grant Market to Exceed $4 Billion in 2000," *CenterWatch*, Vol. 7, Issue 11, November 2000, p. 7.

x Ibid., *CenterWatch*, p. 7.

CHAPTER 2

Expanding Your Physical Space

- Location, Location, Location
- Locating Satellite Offices
- Space Planning
- Lease or Own
- In Review

As your investigative site grows, so too does the need for more physical space. Once the site expands operations beyond an occasional trial or two, the space dedicated to performing clinical trials must be able to handle the flow of study volunteers; offices for study coordinators; visits from monitors, sponsors and FDA auditors; storage of supplies, equipment and study drug; and offer some capability for records retention. A site offering sufficient, clean, modern space to accommodate ongoing studies will project a more professional image to sponsors that are selecting sites, and to patients who spend time at the site during study visits. Having adequate space to conduct clinical trials safely and properly is also a good clinical practice (GCP) guideline.[i]

Palm Beach Research Center (PBRC) started with 1200 square feet of dedicated research space and functioned within that space while conducting ten studies. The site then added 800 square feet. Although this larger 2000-square-foot space seemed adequate at first, we quickly realized that it was still too small for current studies and for our anticipated growth. One year later, when it was time to grow again, we opted to stay in our great location and expand sideways into the adjacent suite, adding 1000 square feet.

Our plan was thwarted, however, when the owner of the space reneged on his promise to lease the newly enlarged space to PBRC at the same rate as the smaller space. We discovered this one month prior to the expiration of the lease in the old space when he forwarded a new lease showing a substantial rent increase. This deception turned out to be a blessing in disguise. Because we were unable to negotiate a satisfactory settlement, we moved to larger space on the first floor in the same building and, in the process, gained better exposure.

The new area was 5200 square feet of dedicated research space. After we signed a five-year lease, the space was built out to our specifications. The lease increased our anxiety level and was a good test of our commitment to this business. We considered the space to be excessive for our needs, but we grew into it within two years. Eventually, this space became too small. At that point, we began looking into the addition of satellite locations.

As mentioned in Chapter 1, clinical research is a young industry lacking in specific benchmarks. Consequently, there is no precise or even general formula to calculate adequate square footage for growing sites. When we added satellite offices, we considered several factors (Table 1). Collectively, they provided a hint as to the amount of space we needed. As a general rule, sites conducting eight to ten studies need 500 square feet per study coordinator, assuming the site conducts all or most of its studies at the site. Less space is required if the site plans to conduct mostly hospital-based trials.

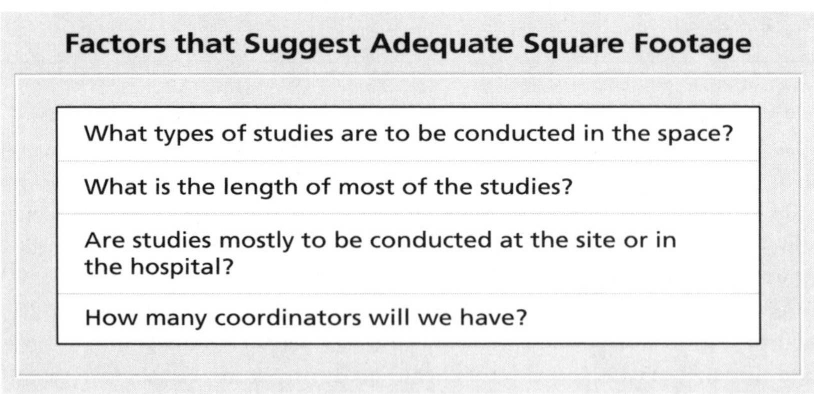

Factors that Suggest Adequate Square Footage
What types of studies are to be conducted in the space?
What is the length of most of the studies?
Are studies mostly to be conducted at the site or in the hospital?
How many coordinators will we have?

Table 1

One space planning issue that can be overlooked by the less experienced investigative site is the fact that studies lasting for several years place an additional burden on the on-site storage capabilities of the site. As long as the study is active, the site will want to keep all of the associated paperwork on hand, instead of sending it to off-site storage. For this reason, it is a good idea to err on the side of too much on-site storage space instead of too little.

We know that some types of studies, such as pharmacokinetic studies, and certain respiratory trials, require more space than others. Pharmacokinetic studies often require blood draws every hour or less for a period of 8 to 24 hours, depending on the protocol. Some respiratory studies, such as asthma or COPD, call for 12-hour visits, which, based on enrollment, can tie up multiple exam rooms and/or the lounge for the entire day.

Studies that are short and require large enrollments can also use lots of space, not to mention parking. For example, trials for over-the-counter (OTC) pain medicine, or for wounds resulting in simple scrapes can easily enroll 100 to 200 participants. Simple studies with limited enrollment, such as those targeting diabetes, hypertension and arthritis, are generally less space-intensive as patient visits last approximately one hour.

Location, Location, Location

By situating the site next to busy medical practices or medical office buildings, or even in a hospital, the site has increased its chances for success. Patient recruitment can be facilitated because there is already a steady flow of patient traffic. The best way to develop awareness of the site is to notify the physicians in the medical office buildings and to specify the types of studies you can conduct. You may consider recruiting some of the physicians as investigators to gain access to their patient populations and to allay fears that your site will steal their patients.

One of the larger sites in our area recently downsized. It initially had a large facility on the edge of town. After a reduction in personnel, the site relocated into a medical office building that was next door to a busy, four-doctor primary care practice. The site formed an association with the senior doctor and, as a result, has accelerated recruitment efforts for all of its studies.

During the site location process, demographics must be taken into consideration. How heavily populated is your geographic area of interest? Are retirement communities nearby? What about hotels and restaurants for visiting monitors or company representatives? How accessible is the airport?

One of the larger trial site companies uses a simple system to establish its offices. It locates sites next to or in close proximity to busy shopping malls. This affords great traffic flow and quick access to food courts, a factor that can be important when volunteers have unusually long study visits. Typically, these sites are successful. This is an approach used by many fast food chains. Some try to locate as close as possible to new McDonald's restaurants, assuming that if McDonald's selected a specific area, it must be a good location.[ii] A younger site can use this same tactic. It can locate near a large, established site that is known to be successful.

One investigator in the Southwest used a slightly different method. He specializes in diabetes studies and located his site in an area with a heavy Hispanic population. According to the American Diabetes Association, the prevalence of Type 2 diabetes is two times higher in Hispanics than in non-Hispanic whites.[iii] His site was immediately successful and it remains a top enroller in diabetes studies.

Locating Satellite Offices

As the site becomes more established, the investigator may consider opening satellite locations. Many investigative sites in large cities can benefit by expanding into different neighborhoods. This type of growth offers access to new populations, and decreases patient travel time to the main site. When investigating the opening of satellite offices, the rule of locating near major shopping centers still applies. Access to major highways and public transportation routes should also be evaluated.

It is worth mentioning that once satellite sites are opened, and sub-investigators are conducting the same studies at those sites that the principal investigator is conducting at the main site, the principal investigator still maintains responsibility for study conduct at the satellite locations.[iv]

Space Planning

Once the space is selected, it is worthwhile to work with a space planner who is familiar with layout and traffic flow in doctors' offices. A space planning professional can help the investigator maximize efficiency in office layout. Many medical office buildings provide space planning services to tenants as part of the lease package. While it is ideal to work with someone who has designed space for other clinical trials' ventures, it is rather unusual to find someone with this experience.

Space planners design layouts typically found in doctors' offices. Other design elements may be unique to clinical research:

- Study coordinators' offices
- Drug supply room
- Records retention and regulatory binder storage room
- Monitor work room
- Laboratory
- Conference room
- Large number of telephone lines and Internet connections, some of which are dedicated for data transmission

Lease or Own

After the decision is made to dedicate space to perform clinical trials, the next decision is whether to lease or own the space. There are pros and cons to both. When a site is expanding for the first time, leasing provides an attractive option because it limits the site's liability to the duration of the lease. If the venture proves to be successful, there may be opportunities to renew the lease and expand within the current location, or the site may opt to relocate once the lease expires. If the site is not successful, there may be ways to terminate the lease before the term is up.

Owning space becomes a more viable alternative once the site has an established presence, affording the site a steady income. A good model for ownership is the medical office building (MOB) option. An MOB gives a site ready access to patients and traffic flow. Bringing this type of project to fruition involves hiring a real estate professional to locate good sites that are available and zoned for an MOB. If a good site is not officially for sale, the real estate agent can approach the owner to learn if he or she would consider selling.

If the land is for sale, the realtor should ask the seller if he or she is willing to give an option to buy the land, which could work as follows: You negotiate an option to buy the land, which lasts for four months. During that time, you perform due diligence to learn specifics about the zoning, such as the size of the building that can fit on the land, presence of on-site utilities, the required parking, setbacks, green space, etc.

Once it is clearly determined that the land can be purchased or optioned, the investigator should plan a meeting with local physicians who are looking to expand their present space or whose leases are expiring. One way to structure deals is to offer the physicians either limited partnerships or long-term leases in the new building where clinical research trials will be conducted in close proximity to their offices, some of which may benefit their patients. Once physicians commit to the project and sign letters of intent, the investigator can use these letters as a form of collateral when seeking financing for the project. Local lenders often look kindly on commercial buildings that attract successful physicians with busy practices. After the option period expires, you can either move forward with the purchase, negotiate to extend the option period or walk away from the deal if the project is less promising than anticipated.

Another route to consider is partnering with the real estate developer, especially if he or she has experience in developing medical office buildings, particularly in your geographic area of choice. If so, that developer will be familiar with idiosyncrasies of that area's zoning and zoning board. By partnering in this way, the developer should be more motivated to do all of the legwork to get the project moving, especially if you provide the names of some interested doctors who want to be limited partners or long-term tenants.

When the project is completed, the real estate professional can act as the leasing agent and property manager as it is the rare doctor who has the time, inclination or know-how to assume all the tasks associated with management of commercial property. If you have difficulty locating a developer, approach your banker and explain your idea. He or she can usually direct you to a reputable realtor or developer to help with your project.

Lines of Credit

Once you make the decision to grow your site, you will need to establish a line of credit from a bank. For newly expanded sites, the reasons for this are basically twofold. First, you will need seed money to pay for the increased staff and possibly larger office space that must be in place before accepting more studies. Secondly, once you discover that slow payments from sponsors and CROs are the rule, you will have realized that your business is probably not generating enough cash to pay existing bills while making expenditures needed for new study startup. For these reasons, a credit line is a necessary evil for growth. If you are conducting one or two studies, the site can be subsidized by your medical practice, but the landscape changes dramatically once you start conducting enough studies to require cash to pay for expanded infrastructure.

The key challenge in establishing a line of credit is that banks generally do not understand the clinical trials business. When applying for a line of credit, it may be helpful to provide a list of your negotiated contracts to specify the revenues your business is and will be generating. An unsecured line of credit is the best choice, but your chances are slim for getting an unsecured line for a new business that banks often do not understand. Even with contracts in hand, and evidence of receivables, you may be asked to guarantee a line of credit personally, using your personal assets as collateral. This is certainly a scary proposition and may discourage many people from taking that step toward site expansion.

A good relationship with the lender increases your chances of obtaining and expanding a line of credit. At first, you may be able to procure only $40,000 to $50,000; however, by returning to the bank periodically with documentation of your site's growing success and increasing revenues, negotiating an increase in the credit line becomes more probable.

Lines of credit are also important for established sites experiencing natural lulls in the business cycle. Down cycles are more likely to occur in midsummer and around the Christmas holiday season. During slow periods, there will be times when you need to tap into your credit line. This tends to be a better choice than laying off personnel to whom you have a commitment. When slow periods hit, training sessions can increase, SOPs can be updated and personnel can give community talks. The time should be used to invest in site improvement activities.

Palm Beach Research Center started by securing a hefty bank loan to build dedicated research space and hire an experienced staff. The early days of PBRC are a good example attesting to the importance of implementing a multi-faceted proactive business development plan. After 18 months of first waiting for studies to come to us and then making some labor-intensive attempts at procuring studies on our own (all the while paying off our bank loan), we realized that we needed to hire a full-time marketing professional. I recommend that you not wait 18 months to do this, but do it as soon as possible after everything you need to do an increased number of studies is in place. I wish I had.

In Review

There is more to expanding operations than hiring additional study coordinators and updating the computer system. A site that is serious about conducting clinical trials must invest in the proper space with the necessary elements. Dedicated research space should have, at the very least, its own entrance, waiting room and exam rooms. Other key elements include space for the study coordinators, monitors, records storage and drug storage. Although there are no industry benchmarks indicating the amount of needed space, a rough guideline is 500 square feet per study coordinator. As the clinical operation grows, space for quality assurance and regulatory professionals should be added, although these additions can mean site expansion or relocation.

When identifying a location for the site, it is critical to consider the demographics of the area of interest, access to major interstates and bus lines, and proximity to eating establishments. There is anecdotal evidence to suggest that locating next to or near major shopping malls can be a good choice because of the steady stream of customers flowing into and out of those areas. Another good location can be into or next to medical office buildings, which not only offer patient traffic, but possible access to physicians who could become sub-investigators.

Finally, when selecting and planning space, the investigator will need to evaluate leasing versus ownership. Most choose to lease space initially to limit the financial obligation and the time dedicated to clinical research. The ownership option can prove lucrative, but investigators choosing this option need to find real estate professionals to handle many, if not most, of the tasks associated with maintaining ownership of a medical office building (MOB). Even if the services of a real estate professional are used, it is still important to be involved, at some level, in the planning stages of the project and in the running of the building. This is simply good business practice.

Ultimately, expanding your space sends a very positive signal to sponsors and CROs. It indicates that the site is successful and that it is established and updating its facilities. Study volunteers who walk into an attractive, modern and clean site are apt to feel more comfortable and less apprehensive about participating in a study.

References

[i] International Conference on Harmonization (ICH) Good Clinical Practice (GCP) guideline 4.2.3.

[ii] *Fast Food Nation*, Eric Schlosser, Houghton Mifflin, 2001, p. 65.

[iii] *http://www.diabetes.org/dar*, accessed June 6, 2001.

[iv] Title 21 Code of Federal Regulations (CFR) 312.53 (g).

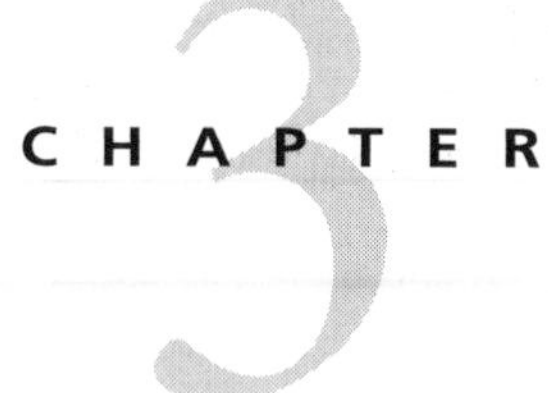

CHAPTER 3

Hiring and Retaining Your Study Coordinators

- Tactics for Keeping Your Study Coordinator
- Don't Forget About Benefits
- Training
- In Review

Study coordinators play such a valuable role that I've devoted this entire chapter to tips on how to retain them and how to recognize when you need more. As your site takes on more studies as it grows, the workload for the study coordinator(s) will grow with it. At some point, even the most efficiently run operation will have harried coordinators, unless the site hires more. At Palm Beach Research Center (PBRC), we have learned to recognize signs of stress exhibited by our coordinators, indicating that they might be overloaded, and it may be time to hire. Some telltale signs are:

- Coordinators are having trouble returning telephone calls in a timely manner.
- Patient visits are so heavily scheduled that there is insufficient time for completion of paperwork.
- Data transmission is behind schedule.
- Monitors start complaining that they are unable to sit with the coordinator for more than a few minutes because the coordinator is continually popping out of the room to tend to something else.
- Coordinators have very little time to see patients in the private practice.

At this stage of our development, PBRC hires coordinators in anticipation of several studies. Sometimes this results in our being temporarily overstaffed, but this situation generally resolves itself when anticipated studies start flowing in. Young sites often make the mistake of procuring a study and then scrambling to find a coordinator. This creates a frenetic environment and puts the site behind the eight ball even before the study begins.

While investigators perform physicals and procedures on the study subjects in accordance with the protocol, they need to recognize that the day-to-day running of the trial is the job of the study coordinator. The timely enrollment of study subjects, the completion of case report forms, proper protocol adherence and the quality of data—critical hands-on elements that define success or failure of the site—are largely the responsibility of the coordinator. The tasks are medical, administrative, regulatory, computer-related, patient-related and marketing-related. Across this broad spectrum, some coordinator responsibilities include:

- Patient recruitment activities
- Completing case report forms
- Scheduling patient visits
- Transmitting study data
- Meeting with monitors
- Meeting with principal investigators
- Shipping samples to laboratories
- Maintaining inventory and accountability of the test item
- Closing out the study
- Participating in preparing proposals for soliciting new studies
- Participating in budget preparation
- Attending investigator meetings

In addition to this list, the coordinator may be doing clerical work, too, depending upon the size of the site and its commitment to a professional environment. The smaller investigative sites may find the coordinator answering telephones, making photocopies and gathering paperwork for study initiation. At PBRC, we have evolved to the point that coordinators can make more productive use of their time than was possible in our earlier years. We have the luxury of an ancillary staff of administrative assistants, research assistants, patient recruiters, regulatory, data and quality assurance personnel who perform many of the tasks that coordinators can be saddled with at growing sites. Our support component frees up the coordinators, allowing them to concentrate on seeing patients, completing the requisite paperwork, doing data submission and the many other activities that require their attention. The goal is to create a professional work environment conducive to more content, less harried coordinators who are better able to produce clean, reliable data.

It is worth noting that even the most nurturing work environment may not prevent the coordinator from pursuing the lure of better paying jobs.

Specifically, experienced study coordinators often see themselves as candidates for more lucrative clinical research associate (monitoring) positions at pharmaceutical, biotechnology or contract research organizations.

Our experience at Palm Beach Research Center has taught us that some study coordinators consider their stint at the investigative site as a training ground for future monitoring positions, especially because both jobs require similar skill sets. In particular, good coordinators and good monitors are Type A personalities who are detail-oriented, compulsive about protocol compliance and focused on proper data collection.

Study coordinators have frequent contact with monitors, so they are in a position to observe and learn specifics of the monitor's job. Once they have mastered certain skills, some coordinators may begin actively searching for monitor positions using traditional job search channels in addition to the Internet and industry conferences. They may also find themselves being pursued by sponsors and CROs. There is more driving this transition than the difference in pay. According to Nancy Ellis, an experienced study coordinator based in South Florida, a key reason why coordinators start searching is that "coordinators are often inundated. If you are detail-oriented, as coordinators have to be, you often lack the time needed to get your work done, especially if the coordinator is responsible for five studies, all at the same time. This causes frustration."

A 1999 survey conducted by the Association of Clinical Research Professionals (ACRP) showed that of the more than 2000 clinical professionals who participated, nearly 50% had changed employers in the preceding three years. Of the various types of professionals represented, 42% of them were coordinators.[i]

Average Annual Salary Growth by Employer

	0–5%	6–10%	11–20%	21%+
Pharma	38.4%	26.9%	17.7%	13.5%
Large CRO	34.1%	23.7%	16.2%	24.9%
Independent Site	56.3%	18.0%	12.4%	11.6%

Table 1 Source: ACRP White Paper 2000

That same survey also revealed several factors about salary growth. First, salary increases at sponsor and CRO venues outpaced those of independent sites (Table 1). Secondly, monitors' salaries were growing faster than other job classifications, with at least one-third of them reporting double-digit pay increases in the preceding three years. By comparison, less than one-quarter of study coordinators reported double-digit pay increases.[ii]

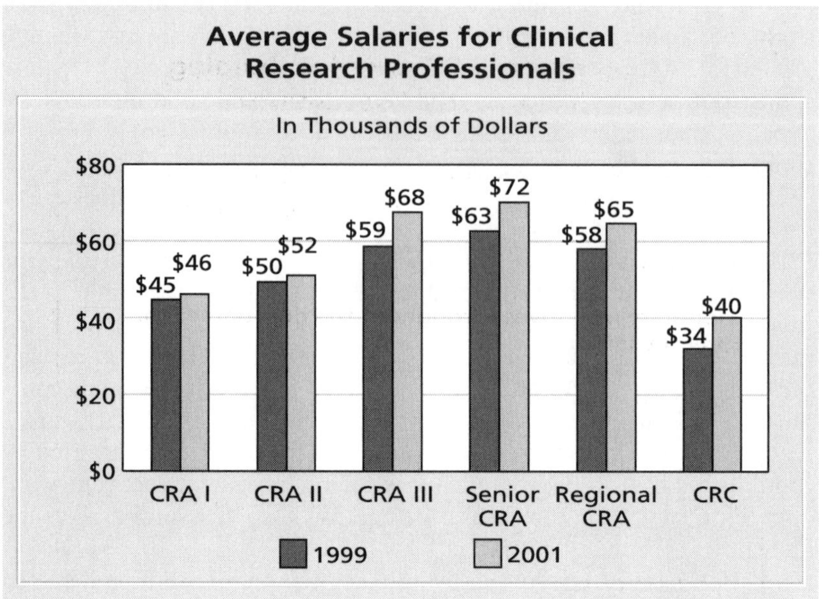

Figure 1 Source: CenterWatch

A 2001 CenterWatch survey of forty-five sponsors, CROs, SMOs and independent sites showed wide disparities between coordinator and monitor salaries.[iii] Whereas beginning monitors earned in the mid-$40K range, advancing to the $60K-plus range for senior monitors,* coordinators were more likely to earn about $40K, and were less likely to have a defined job ladder similar to those available to monitors (Figure 1). Some sites, depending upon their size, do offer advancement opportunities to coordinators. A large site might have a senior coordinator position, followed by a supervisor of clinical operations.

The data revealed in these surveys make it is easy to understand why a coordinator might target a monitoring position as a smart career move.

Tactics for Keeping Your Study Coordinator

Although monitoring positions generally offer greater financial reward and a defined career ladder, monitoring isn't for everybody. Extensive travel is

* Independent monitors can earn more than those employed by sponsors or CROs.

often required, sites may be indifferent or less than cordial to visiting monitors, and they may have to tolerate difficult behavior from investigators who resent being questioned or allocating time to meet with the monitor.

A Summary of Tactics for Keeping Your Study Coordinator
Enable coordinators to maximize patient contact
Time flexibility
Monetary incentives throughout the duration of the clinical trial
Competitive pay
Provide coordinator training
Recognize excellent performance with verbal and written "thank-you's"
Good benefits package
Professional work environment

Table 2

From this perspective, the coordinator's job looks more enticing. Site management can take steps to enhance the job further. First and foremost, management needs to recognize that many coordinators place a high value on the patient contact afforded by clinical research. Being able to interact with and observe patients who are participating in cutting-edge clinical research are activities that many coordinators particularly enjoy. By comparison, a monitor's job affords virtually no patient contact.

At PBRC we seek coordinators who make patient contact a priority. Often, they are nurses with various backgrounds or other types of ancillary personnel who enjoy patient contact. We have found that coordinators who like working with patients are more likely to stay if they have lots of patient interaction and if they feel the site emphasizes the well-being of the patients. This type of person may be less likely to seek a monitoring position once he or she recognizes that monitors have minimal patient contact.

Time flexibility may be the most important asset that a site can offer to a coordinator. Enabling a coordinator to arrange his or her schedule to meet the demands of work and family may go a long way toward retaining a coordinator. In the 2001 CenterWatch survey of forty-five sponsors, CROs, SMOs and independent sites, 42% of respondents stated that time flexibility was the key strategy for slowing turnover (Figure 2).

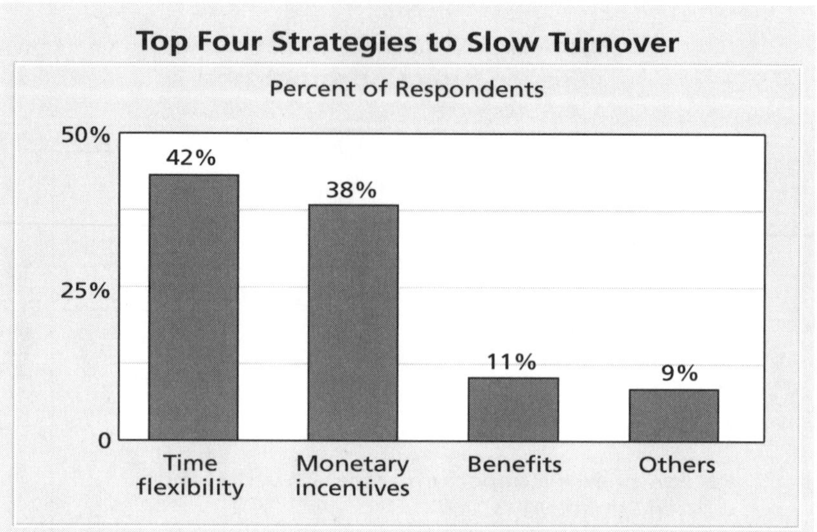

Figure 2 Source: CenterWatch, 2001

Lynne Merriam, president and CEO of Clinical Research of West Florida, agrees that time flexibility is high on the list of coordinator retention strategies. "We are very family-friendly and this makes a big difference. We know that coordinators have family issues that come up, so we make allowances for what people need to do." Merriam also comments that coordinators seeking a flexible, family-friendly environment often have little or no interest in jobs with constant travel. "I've become more astute at hiring. We try to hire people who are not looking at this job as a stepping stone to becoming a monitor. We ask applicants about their long-term goals and determine whether they want to do the heavy traveling that is required of a monitor. Often people with children aren't interested in becoming monitors because of the traveling."

The CenterWatch survey pinpointed improved monetary incentives as the second most important retention method. Respondents identified three key areas in this category:

- Bonuses (58% of respondents)
- Stock Options (25% of respondents)
- Salary Increases (17% of respondents)

It is worth noting that salary increases scored last as monetary incentive. The survey showed that desire for bonuses ranked substantially higher, suggesting that people respond to recognition of their efforts through a bonus reward. This is more coveted than straight salary increases, which institutions sometimes grant to both effective and ineffective coordinators through annual pay raises. A study by the National Science Foundation of 300 cases of productivity, pay and job satisfaction found compelling evidence that compensation based on performance yields higher motivation, productivity and job satisfaction. Data suggested that using a combination of performance, feedback and incentives increased productivity an average of 63.8%.[iv]

A performance-based recognition system can be implemented at the investigative site to recognize coordinators and other team members whose work contributes directly to study success.

A word about teamwork is in order. Although the study coordinator is the key driving force behind study completion, protocol compliance and study success, he or she doesn't do it alone. Studies are generally conducted by a team, especially at larger sites. And recognizing this team is vital. Management theory suggests that reserving rewards for a select few is probably the single greatest mistake that companies make in developing reward systems, particularly in an endeavor that requires teamwork.[v] It's important to recognize everyone involved. This is motivating and enhances *esprit de corps*.

Giving a simple "thank you" can be done either verbally, by email or in writing. Copies of email and written communications should be forwarded to the coordinator's boss or supervisor, and should be placed in the coordinator's employment folder. While thanking staff for a job well done is a common-sense tactic, research suggests that it happens much too infrequently.[vi] One study showed that a personal thank you from the manager and written thanks from the manager were the top two workplace incentives. That same study revealed that 58% of employees reported that they seldom, if ever, receive personal thanks, and 76% said that they seldom, if ever, received written praise.

Carmella Ramnes, Research Administrator of the Cancer Center at Albany Medical College says she thanks her coordinators daily for their efforts. Also, she frequently bakes, gives Christmas gifts and makes greeting cards for her staff.

PBRC gives verbal recognition at Friday meetings by announcing any exceptional work efforts from the previous week. At the end of studies, recognition certificates are presented publicly to coordinators for outstanding performance.

One study coordinator for a small regional SMO stated that her company does not recognize coordinators at all. They are never thanked verbally or in writing or made to feel valuable in any way. In fact, her company's organizational chart places coordinators at the bottom of the chart, below the administrative assistants. Training is not provided beyond a quick ninety-minute overview, and coordinators are routinely blamed if enrollment targets are not met. Even though the company pays an excellent salary, and the coordinators have good time flexibility, the lack of recognition and professional respect contributes to a heavy turnover.

Don't Forget About Benefits

Retaining the coordinator requires multiple strategies and goes beyond raising the base pay. While recognition is certainly key, so too is an appropriate benefits package. The CenterWatch survey identified several areas to be improved (Figure 3).

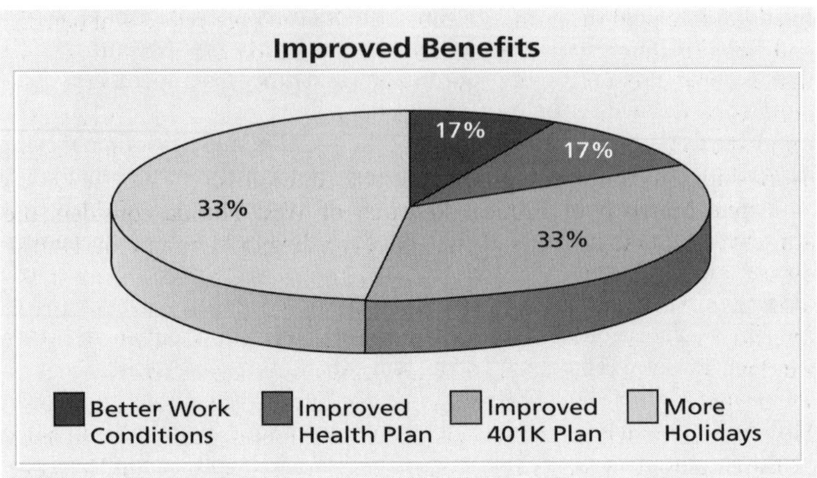

Figure 3 Source: CenterWatch, 2001

The goal is to create an attractive package that makes it difficult for coordinators to consider a job change. Ideally, the package should be a combination of financial, vacation and quality-of-life benefits, and include as many of the following benefits as possible:

- Paid vacation
- Paid holidays
- Health insurance
- Dental insurance
- 401K
- Profit sharing
- Overtime pay

One institution that offers a generous benefits package is Albany Medical College. In addition to health insurance, a prescription program, a dental insurance option, a retirement plan, a tax-deferred annuity and a tuition reimbursement program, there is a good vacation plan. This package includes 24 to 30 personal days annually, which is a combination of vacation plus sick time. There are six additional paid holidays plus one more designated holiday every six months. "If you don't use all of the personal days each year, they can be banked, up to 150 days. This is for anyone who works at

Albany Medical College, not just the coordinators," says Carmella Ramnes. In addition, the college has worked hard to create positive working conditions for all staff. Albany Medical College affords its staff flexible hours, on-site daycare facilities, an on-site bank, dry-cleaning services, an on-site travel agency, discount tickets to some local events and an excellent cafeteria.

While independent sites are not positioned to offer the sorts of benefits found at large academic medical centers, they can still offer a good package. In addition to paid vacation, sick time, health insurance, retirement benefits and flex-time, independent sites can offer profit sharing and bonus plans that are linked to productivity. Academic medical centers tend not to offer bonuses, viewing them as a conflict-of-interest. The more entrepreneurial-minded coordinators working at independent sites will enjoy the sense of ownership that comes with productivity-based rewards.

Lynne Merriam of Clinical Research of West Florida considers the attractive facility to be a definite benefit. According to Merriam, this family-owned independent site located on a one-acre wooded lot has the most up-to-date medical equipment, telephone system, computers and high-speed Internet access. Each coordinator has his or her own private office with a window. Merriam comments, "The coordinators' offices are their own personal space. This creates a sense of professionalism and autonomy." Merriam's approach confirms what research has found, namely that high up on the employees' wish list are an enjoyable work environment and a feeling that they're making an impact in their jobs.[vii]

Training

Nothing speaks to a site's commitment to its staff like investing in their training. Not only is training the best way to teach coordinators about the many federal guidelines overseeing clinical research, it also sends a signal that the site seeks to create a professional workplace of trained employees. Sponsors and CROs involved in site selection are bound to look more favorably on sites with a stable, trained staff because the expectation is that they are better prepared than those without training to enroll patients in a timely fashion, conduct research trials in a compliant manner and capture clean data. At the very least, training should serve to reduce the number of queries generated during data cleanup. Metrics suggest that a single error costs $80 to $150 to correct, translating into billions of dollars spent annually to clean up data from sites.[viii]

A 1999 ACRP survey of more than 2000 of its members showed that 76% of them ranked the need to train study coordinators as the most important area of training.[ix] Coordinators must have a broad knowledge base of regulations such as those spelled out in the various parts of 21 Code of Federal Regulations and the International Code of Harmonization. They also need to be familiar with a range of tasks such as study initiation, methods to enhance patient recruitment initiatives, source documentation, document storage and retrieval and more.

Conveying this information to the coordinator requires a mix of formal and informal training followed by ongoing education in the form of inservices, workshops, seminars, conferences and mentoring. The site's willingness to invest in this training indicates its respect for the professional status of the coordinator. Inexperienced coordinators who are not trained, or are trained in a slipshod, on-the-job manner will have little knowledge of their responsibilities and may feel overwhelmed by the volume of paperwork and endless details of study conduct they are expected to handle. It is easy to understand how this can result in feelings of frustration and alienation, and lead to a high rate of turnover.

The Association of Clinical Research Professionals (ACRP) and the Society of Clinical Research Associates (SoCRA) offer training courses as well as examinations leading to certification. In order to sit for the certification examination, applicants need either two years of full-time work experience in clinical research, four years of part-time work (ACRP) or 3,500 hours over the past five years (SoCRA). Continuing education is required by both bodies to maintain certification. Sites with high professional standards often encourage their coordinators to become certified, and typically pay for the dues and the courses needed for certification. In addition, they often pay for the continuing education courses required to maintain the certification.

In Review

The smart site aiming to retain its study coordinators will take a multifaceted approach. This includes enabling the coordinator to have lots of patient contact and offering flexible work schedules, training, monetary incentives, performance bonuses, health insurance, paid vacations, paid holidays and retirement plans. There should also be formal and informal ways of recognizing employees for their contributions. Once these programs are in place, the hope is that the site will have created an atmosphere that is too attractive for coordinators to contemplate leaving.

Merriam of Clinical Research of West Florida offers a competitive salary along with a package of benefits and a positive, attractive working environment that has resulted in three of her eleven coordinators staying with her since 1995, the year the company started. Other coordinators added as the company expanded have stayed, too, except those who have relocated to other parts of the country. Merriam attributes her strong record of keeping coordinators to the professional atmosphere and a genuine, almost familial, caring about her employees.

At PBRC, the efforts to create a positive working environment have paid off handsomely. Since we instituted motivation and recognition programs, such as bonuses for reaching study milestones, verbal recognition at Friday meetings and recognition certificates at the end of studies, we have retained our coordinators for lengthy periods and have experienced little turnover. We also keep a sharp eye out for coordinator overload, indicating that we may need to hire more. Prior to implementing these efforts, most of our coordinators quit after a six- to twelve-month stint.

Although there do not seem to be any formal surveys looking specifically at the impact of work environment on coordinator retention, there is anecdotal evidence. A CenterWatch article on study coordinator retention looks at what sites, SMOs and academic medical centers can offer to coordinators.[x] Representatives from the three venues generally recognize the importance of good benefits, flex-time arrangements and training, yet each environment offers unique advantages that could boost coordinator retention. Coordinators at academic medical centers may be drawn to the prestige of research institutions and the opportunity to work with key opinion leaders. Those at smaller sites may like the ability to interact freely with top decision makers and may enjoy the minimal bureaucracy that characterizes small sites. SMOs look to coordinators to play a major role in assuring quality across multiple sites. To help coordinators be successful in this role, SMO management may invest in coordinator training programs that include a standard curriculum plus a review of company-wide SOPs. According to the article, good programs go a long way toward retaining coordinators, but SMOs seem to be the most vulnerable to losing coordinators to monitoring positions.[xi]

Retaining the study coordinator will be one of the biggest challenges for the growing site. Acknowledging that benefits and flex-time are important, that ongoing recognition and bonuses are motivating and that coordinators want and need training can help a site design programs to improve coordinator retention. These programs are most successful when the site applies them to appropriate candidates, ideally those who enjoy patient contact and are disinterested in the heavy travel associated with higher paying monitoring positions. Surveys have identified these two elements as the key reasons that coordinators give for not jumping to monitoring positions. Professional respect, a reasonable workload and competitive pay also figure heavily into retention strategies.

References

[i] "Where we are and where we're going," *The Monitor*, Association of Clinical Research Professionals, James W. Maloy et al., Summer 2000, p. 18.

[ii] Ibid., "Where we are and where we're going," p. 24.

[iii] "Evolving Employment Trends in the Clinical Trials Industry," DIA Annual Meeting 2001, Joan A. Kroll, CenterWatch; Marianne Considine, Advanced Clinical Services.

[iv] *Second to None, How Our Smartest Companies Put People First*, Charles Garfield, Business One Irwin, 1992, p. 250.

[v] Ibid., *Second to None, How Our Smartest Companies Put People First*, p. 258.

[vi] *The Employee Recruitment and Retention Handbook*, Diane Arthur, American Management Association, 2001, pp. 33-34.

[vii] *The Employee Recruitment and Retention Handbook*, Diane Arthur, American Management Association, 2001, p. 33.

[viii] "Clinical Research in Transition," *The Monitor*, Association of Clinical Research Professionals, James W. Maloy et al., Summer 2001, Vol. 15, Issue 2, p. 31.

[ix] "Where we are and where we're going," *The Monitor*, Association of Clinical Research Professionals, James W. Maloy et al., Summer 2000, p. 25.

[x] "Don't Let Your Study Coordinator Get Away," *CenterWatch*, September 1, 1998, Amy Tsao, Vol. 9, Issue 9.

[xi] Ibid., "Don't Let Your Study Coordinator Get Away," p. 15.

CHAPTER

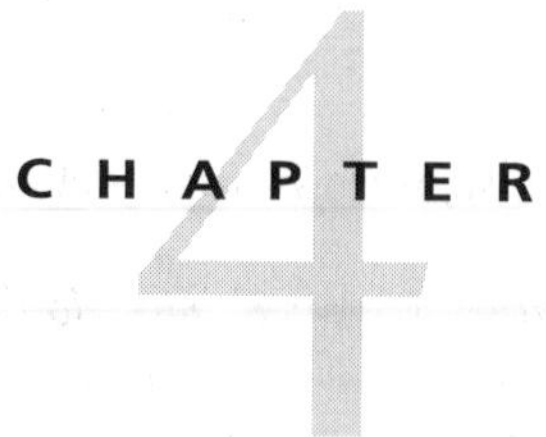

Operations and Quality Assurance Personnel and Procedures

- Director of Clinical Operations
- Quality Assurance
- Data Management
- Regulatory Affairs
- A Few Comments About Audits
- Inspections by Sponsors
- In Review

If a site is to grow successfully, specific functions of the clinical trials process must first be solidly in place. A common pitfall in this industry is for the owner to promote his or her investigative site before it can adequately perform more studies. This happens when site management has not yet recognized the critical importance of developing the appropriate infrastructure needed to support the site aiming to grow its clinical trials business carefully and thoughtfully.

The areas discussed in this chapter are basic functions needed to build a firm foundation for growth with quality.

Director of Clinical Operations (DCO)

The Director of Clinical Operations (DCO) is crucial to site growth and, assuming the right person is hired, will be instrumental in moving the site to the next level. The DCO oversees all of the day-to-day clinical operations. He or she meets weekly with all study coordinators; assigns studies to the study coordinators based on their experience and current workload; participates in all study initiations, close-out meetings, monitor visits, FDA and sponsor audits; meets with the quality assurance team to discuss trends and issues; acts as a liaison between the sponsor, investigator and study coordinator to address issues relating to protocol compliance; oversees formal staff training; and is involved in any clinically related issue with regard to budgeting, contracting and salary reviews. The DCO is the glue that holds the site together. All study coordinators, research assistants, regulatory staff and laboratory personnel report to the DCO, who then reports directly to the principal investigator and the CEO.

The ideal candidate is someone who has had site experience, is familiar with good clinical practice standards and has a clinical background, such as a nurse who has worked in an ICU or in some other type of nursing environment with rigid, military-like rules and constraints. Hiring someone with this kind of background will increase the likelihood that the individual can function in a highly structured, regulated workplace. The DCO should also have management and leadership skills. Previous experience as a monitor is desirable, but it is strongly preferred that the DCO have site experience as a study coordinator, or as some other site-based clinical professional.

Recruiting a DCO is a challenge. Because of the importance of this position—and the impact it will have on the site's growth—it is recommended that the DCO be someone who is known to you or is referred to you by a trusted source.

Example 1 – Selecting the wrong person for DCO and the consequences

A large site was excited about its growth and decided that it was time to hire a DCO. Jim, who had worked in the industry, was hired. He had started out as a scientist and eventually became quite successful in bench research and in the laboratory. He had exemplary credentials and had worked for a CRO. The site director was delighted at the prospect of Jim's assuming many of the duties that would contribute to the site's continued growth. In addition, Jim received accolades from the principal investigator, the site director and the marketing department, all of whom were impressed with his credentials and in-depth knowledge of the industry.

Unfortunately, from the get-go, there were little signs that were not heeded by management. Jim started altering simple standard operating procedures (SOPs) that had worked very well. One example is that he altered the method for reporting adverse events and serious adverse advents. He also took over many tasks that had been successfully handled by the study coordinators and assumed those responsibilities himself. With his time being so consumed with the many duties involved in running daily clinical trials, plus overseeing the study coordinators and his other responsibilities, he was unable to do any of his tasks efficiently. The whole system broke down.

Complaints from monitors, sponsors and CROs poured into the site, which was widely regarded to be among the top sites in the country. The site director was completely disheartened and had to eventually sit down with Jim and separate the tasks. Jim left the organization, eventually joining a medium-sized CRO where he did quite well. The parting was both professional and congenial.

The lessons that everyone learned from this is that Jim knew the industry and the CRO side of the business, but that this knowledge did not translate into his having the management experience or an understanding of operations at the site level. The site director learned that a successful DCO needs to have site-level experience, particularly in site management.

Quality Assurance

The growing site needs to establish a quality assurance (QA) department, even if that department starts with nothing more than a single full-time equivalent (FTE) or a part-time resource, depending upon workload. A number of site alliances and site management organizations (SMOs) share one quality assurance FTE who travels from site to site to QA the charts prior to monitor visits. Sponsors, CROs and monitors recognize and appreciate this investment in quality.

The purpose of the QA department is to develop and implement programs designed to improve the quality of studies conducted at the site,[i] starting from day one. This raises the bar for patient safety and should enhance outcomes of monitoring visits. Key responsibilities of the QA department are listed in Table 1.

The QA function is a standard business practice for overseeing product quality. Quality assurance, as defined by the International Standardization Organization (ISO 9000), refers to planned and systematic activities necessary to provide adequate confidence that a product or service will satisfy requirements for quality.[ii]

Applying this definition to the clinical trials industry, QA serves to ensure that Good Clinical Practice (GCP) guidelines are adhered to, resulting in a quality product, which, in this case, is a well-run clinical trial that produces clean, reliable data. According to the Food and Drug Administration, GCP is an international ethical and scientific quality standard for designing, conducting, recording and reporting of trials that involve the participation of human subjects. Compliance with this standard provides assurance that the rights, safety and well-being of study subjects are protected, consistent with the principles originating with the Declaration of Helsinki, and that the clinical trial data are credible.[iii] The guidelines spell out responsibilities for the investigator, the investigational review board (IRB) and the sponsor.

Key Responsibilities of the Quality Assurance Department
Compliance with Good Clinical Practice (GCP)
Compliance with FDA regulations
Compliance with the site's standard operating procedures (SOPs)
Compliance with protocol requirements such as inclusion/exclusion criteria, performance of required procedures, visits made within protocol-required windows and other tasks
Review of all tracking forms prior to study initiation
Review of 100% of the informed consent forms and the consent verification logs
Review source documentation, encompassing a minimum of 10% of patient charts in all active studies, using a defined turnaround time for chart review, such as 8, 24 or 72 hours
Look for trends/discrepancies in documentation and review problems with the Director of Clinical Operations to correct and prevent future errors

Table 1

Conducting trials in a GCP-compliant manner is a tall order, requiring that investigators be trained in the many aspects of proper trial conduct and that sites complete and maintain various types of study-related documentation. The QA department is a natural fit to manage training of and compliance with these GCP-related activities.

Because of its importance, the QA team should report to the highest level of management and maintain independence from the operations group.[iv] In addition, the QA team should be presented to the site as a positive, cooperative force and not as adversarial to site operations.[v] Using this approach, the QA team can audit studies at prescribed times, such as at study startup, and once a month thereafter. Findings of each audit are to be shared with the principal investigator, sub-investigators, study coordinators and any other personnel involved with the study. The auditing exercise can serve to prepare the site for monitoring visits, FDA audits and sponsor audits. A sample visit checklist appears in the Appendix. In addition, the QA department can provide monitors with an evaluation form to be completed at the conclusion of the visit. The completed form will provide direction for the site and will highlight areas needing improvement. This is a useful tool because monitors generally do not share the results of their visits with sites.

To facilitate the operation of a GCP-compliant site, a good QA department works with all levels of management to develop standard operating procedures (SOPs). These procedures are designed to bring consistency to common practices conducted at the site by providing a standard format,

Study Management SOPs
Telephone Screening
Sign-in Sheet
Schedule Book
Confirming Appointments
Informed Consent Process
Amended Consents
Screen Failures
Tracking Forms
Serious Adverse Events
Master Charts
Source Documents
Progress Notes
Obtaining Medical Records, Notifying Primary Care Physician
Storage of Records
Patient Stipend

Table 2

method, authorization trail and implementation process. The goal of SOPs is to improve quality by preventing or limiting errors and non-compliance problems at the site level. The QA department should review the SOPs annually to keep them current and should be diligent about their being followed. A word of warning: If a site has SOPs that are not being followed, an FDA inspector who detects this during an audit is likely to issue a violation (see Section "A Few Comments About Audits").

SOPs address a wide range of clinical and administrative topics, ranging from obtaining informed consent to randomization procedures to collecting data to handling a code on a patient. Some types of "Study Management" SOPs appear in Table 2. Most procedural errors occur with the first three or four patients enrolled in a study; it is a good idea to develop an SOP instructing the QA department to review and approve all charts and source documents for the first four patients in all studies. Once enrollment extends beyond the first few patients, it is suggested to have all paperwork completed by the study coordinator, research assistant or data entry staff within 24 hours of each patient visit. This process limits the number of missed procedures. For example, the study coordinator may have taken a blood pressure reading during the patient visit, and may have quickly jotted

Sample Format for Standard Operating Procedures (SOPs)

Sample Format for Standard Operating Procedures (SOPs)
Title of SOP–Brief description using few words.
Objective–Define the purpose of the SOP and describe why the activity is being done (e.g., to meet GCP guidelines or IRB requirements).
Applicable to–List who needs to follow this SOP.
Definitions–Define any terms used in the SOP, if needed (if none, state, "None").
Related SOPs–List of any other SOPs referenced within this SOP (if none, state, "None").
Procedures–Describe tasks or procedures in a step-by-step fashion. Identify each task/step, naming the person responsible for completing it.
Attachments–Attach sample forms, checklists or other supplemental information, if required.

Table 3

it down on a piece of paper instead of recording it in the case report form. Implementing this simple procedure can improve the quality of the paperwork completed at the site.

Whether sites create their own SOPs, or customize templated SOPs, it is suggested that they include information described in Table 3. A sample SOP appears in Table 4. As added protection it is also suggested that anyone at the site who is given a copy of the SOPs must sign an agreement confirming he or she has received and reviewed them.

Data Management

Data management refers to the process of transferring information from the source documents into case report forms. It does not involve manipulating the data in any way. After the data manager transfers the data, it is the responsibility of the study coordinator to transmit the data to the CRO or sponsor.

Data management is an administrative function, not a clinical one. To simplify the process, it is recommended that the paperwork be lined up in front of the data manager, along with the necessary documentation forms spelling out exactly what information goes where on which form. A sample form could be created for this purpose. This simplifies what can be a tedious job and reduces the incidence of errors. (See the Data Management form in Appendix a.) A research assistant who is well organized and detail-oriented is a good choice for this position. Oftentimes, a medical assistant is successful in this role.

When a site grows to the point that it can justify adding a full-time or part-time data manager, this should result in study coordinators being freed up to schedule and conduct more patient visits and interact in a less pressured way with monitors, investigators and representatives of the sponsor and CRO. This improves the working atmosphere at the site, especially for the study coordinators, which facilitates improved site performance.

It is worth noting that the clinical trials industry has many electronic solutions to data capture and transmission available to it. Even so, the transition is slow and piecemeal, and the majority of studies are still conducted with pen and paper. (See "Electronic Medical Records and Other E-Solutions.") The growing site will continue to need a data manager to transcribe information onto the many paper forms used to document clinical research activity. As data management transitions toward an electronic mode, the role of the data manager will change if source data are collected and transmitted by the study coordinator and investigator during the patient visit, possibly through the use of handheld personal digital assistants (PDAs) or electronic tablets.

Sample SOP–Informed Consent Process

The process by which a subject voluntarily confirms his or her willingness to participate in a particular trial, after having been informed of all aspects of the trial that are relevant to the subject's decision to participate.

Objective: Informed consent is documented by means of a written, signed and dated informed consent form. The SOP has as a regulatory basis: 21 CFR 50.20; 21 CFR 50.27; 45 CFR 46.116; 45 CFR 46.117; GCP Guideline Part 4.8; and FDA Information Sheets for IRBs and Clinical Investigators.

Applicable to: Principal investigator, QA department, regulatory affairs, study coordinator.

Procedure: After patient fills out the registration data and reads the Informed Consent Form (ICF), he/she is given the opportunity to read and review the ICF thoroughly with the study coordinator and/or investigator.

The patient is given an opportunity to ask questions.

The patient is given the option to take a copy of the ICF home to share with family and primary care physician.

After the patient has complete understanding and agrees to participate, the ICF is signed and dated by the patient.

Patient receives a copy of the completed and dated ICF (21 CFR 50.27) and registration data. The original signed ICF is filed with the source documents.

The ICF will then be signed and dated by the person who conducted the informed consent process and/or the investigator.

The site may request from the IRB that an investigator's signature not be required on the ICF. If the investigator's signature is required, it will mean that he or she is either:

1. Confirming an adequate consent process and/or
2. Consenting the patient himself or herself and/or
3. Witnessing the patient's and coordinator's signature process

If the ICF is not signed, no study procedures are to be initiated.

The consent process is documented in the source documents.

Table 4 Source: Ruth Ann Nylen, Ph.D. 2001

Regulatory Affairs

Growth at the site level is accompanied by a tremendous increase in regulatory paperwork generated in support of clinical studies. This workload becomes particularly noticeable once the site reaches a milestone of somewhere between seven and nine ongoing trials. As long as the site participates in a smaller number of trials, it is usually possible to have regulatory responsibilities assumed by an administrator or by the study coordinator. Once this milestone is reached, however, the site will probably need to hire a regulatory affairs person.

Initially, this individual may assume other administrative duties if he or she is not fully consumed with regulatory paperwork, but eventually the position will expand to full-time. Some of the responsibilities of the regulatory affairs person (or eventually, the regulatory affairs director) include corresponding with local, central and in-hospital Institutional Review Boards (IRBs); maintaining all paperwork for the regulatory binder; proper reporting of adverse events (AEs) and serious adverse events (SAEs); and more, as detailed in Table 5. The regulatory affairs department's main goal is to conform to the many guidelines of the National Institutes of Health (NIH) and the Food and Drug Administration (FDA) that govern performance of clinical studies for drugs, biologics, devices and food.

Some of the Tasks Assumed by Regulatory Affairs
Completing regulatory submissions to IRBs, sponsors and CROs
Maintaining all paperwork for the Regulatory Binder
Maintaining PI and sub-PI credentials
Obtaining approvals from IRBs for patient recruitment initiatives
Collaborating with the Quality Assurance Department to prepare for FDA and sponsor audits of the site

Table 5

Dedicating an FTE to regulatory activities will accomplish two major goals: It will free up the study coordinator to perform other study-related tasks and, secondly, it will improve the site's turnaround time for submitting paperwork needed to start up a study. Offering good turnaround time is an important marketing tool for the site. It shows efficiency and complements the skill, knowledge and experience that a site can offer to sponsors. Efficiency is more than a measure of how quickly the site submits a regulatory package. Efficiency is about doing the job correctly the first time and in a timely fashion.

Example 1 – An Organized Regulatory Department Can Help the Site Procure Studies

Several years ago, Palm Beach Research Center (PBRC) was late in learning about a large vaccine trial. Once we did learn about it, we contacted the CRO managing the study to express our interest. The CRO inspected our site and subsequently offered a contract to be a replacement site if any of their already selected research centers fell behind on enrollment. Prior to the investigators' meeting, our site learned from the sponsor's regulatory department that PBRC was the only site that had already completed and submitted all regulatory documents associated with the study. Armed with this information, I communicated with the sponsor's project manager at the investigator's meeting, stating our interest in becoming an original site, and not a replacement site, especially since all of our regulatory documents were in order and submitted ahead of all other sites selected for the study. Upon my return from the investigators' meeting, the study coordinator informed me that PBRC had been picked as an original site. Not only did PBRC do well with the study, but the site also received two additional study extensions over a four-year period.

The regulatory affairs department will necessarily increase in size to keep pace with the needs of a growing site and can emerge as a major resource for the site. A good department can function as a liaison between the various clinical partners: IRBs, sponsors, SMOs, CROs and PIs. Eventually, the cost of this function per site can be spread out if the regulatory department services other sites within a network.

The Regulatory Binder

The regulatory binder is the record of study documentation. Because all clinical studies tend to have many of the same components, the regulatory affairs department, with input from the site, should consider developing a format for the binder that standardizes needed documents for all studies. Although various sponsors and CROs may provide study binders, it is preferable that the site use its own standard binder. This will regiment the site and enhance quality by organizing paperwork needed for proper study conduct and for visits from monitors, the Food and Drug Administration (FDA) and sponsors.

The binder includes:

- IRB-approved signed informed consent forms
- Serious Adverse Event (SAE) reports

- FDA Statement of Investigator Form 1572
- Continuing and final review reports
- CVs and medical licenses of the principal investigator(s) and sub-investigator(s)
- Letters of indemnification and confidentiality
- 21 CFR (Code of Federal Regulations) 54 Financial Disclosure by Clinical Investigators
- Clinical supplies: Proof of receipt of CRFs, lab kits, diaries, etc.
- Protocols, protocol amendments and signature pages
- Investigator brochures
- Drug accountability records
- Telephone logs
- IRB-approved materials, IRB correspondence and Continuing Review Reports
- IRB protocol
- ICF approval letter
- Advertisements and approvals
- General correspondence with the CRO and/or sponsor (includes newsletters)
- Reorder forms
- Site signature and delegation logs (stating who is responsible for which study activity. The logs are signed and initialed.)
- Follow-up forms
- Monitoring logs and reports
- Shipment records
- Screening logs (documenting who was screened for enrollment)
- Laboratory certificates and values
- Equipment logs
- IND safety reports

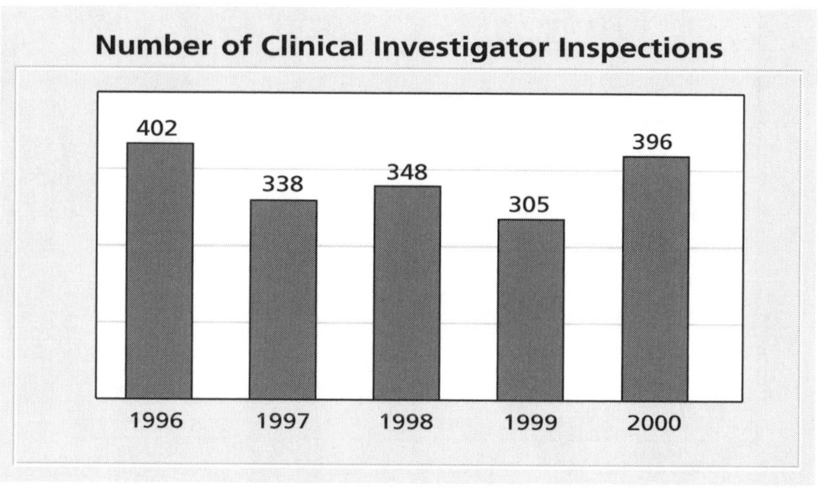

Figure 1

Source: CDER

The real test of your site's preparedness is how it fares during an audit by the Food and Drug Administration (FDA). It's not a question of whether an FDA audit will happen, it's a question of when. According to the Center for Drug Evaluation and Research (CDER), a division of the FDA, there are approximately 400 on-site inspections annually (Figure 1). Inspections can last anywhere from several days for routine inspections to a few weeks if serious problems are uncovered.

Through its Bioresearch Monitoring Program, the FDA carries out three types of clinical investigator audits:[vi]

- Study-Oriented Inspection
- Investigator-Oriented Inspection
- Bioequivalence Study Inspection

The Two Parts of the Study-Oriented Inspection

Facts Surrounding the Conduct of the Study	Auditing of Study Data
Who did what	The inspector compares the data submitted to the Agency and/or sponsor with all available records that might support data
Degree of delegation of authority	The inspector may also review records covering a reasonable period after completion of the study to determine if there was proper follow-up
Where specific aspects of the study were performed	
How and where data were recorded	
How test article (drug) accountability was maintained	
How the monitor communicated with the clinical investigator	
How the monitor evaluated the study's progress	

Table 6 Source: FDA Office of Compliance

The first two types, study- and investigator-oriented, make up the majority of inspections at the investigative site. A study-oriented inspection occurs almost exclusively to review trials that are important to new drug applications (NDAs) or product license applications (PLAs) pending before the agency. This type of study consists of two basic parts—determining the facts surrounding the conduct of the study and an auditing of the study data (Table 6).

The investigator-oriented inspection may occur because an investigator conducted a pivotal study that merits in-depth examination due to its importance in product approval or its effect on medical practice.[vii] This type of inspection may also be initiated for cause. For example, sponsor representatives may have reported to the FDA that it is having difficulty getting case report forms from the investigator, or there is some other concern with the investigator's work. Additional reasons for an investigator-oriented inspection appear in Table 7.

Additional Reasons for an Investigator-Oriented Inspection
A clinical investigator has participated in a large number of studies or has done work outside his or her specialty area
Safety or effectiveness findings are inconsistent with those of other investigators conducting the same study
Too many subjects with a specific disease given the locale of the investigator are claimed
A study subject complains about protocol or subject rights violations
Laboratory results are outside the range of the biological variance

Table 7 Source: Office of FDA Compliance

Whether the inspection is study-oriented or investigator-oriented, a well-organized, well-maintained regulatory binder can show the inspector that all aspects of the study in question are in proper order. Although the clinical investigator is responsible for the conduct of the study and is accountable for the results, maintaining the regulatory binder is the responsibility of the site's regulatory department.

According to the FDA, its inspectors are to pay particular attention to documents with missing dates, times and information. They are also to read X-rays, EKGs and lab results instead of merely recording their presence.[viii] A regulatory affairs department that is aware of what inspectors will be looking for can develop the regulatory binder to facilitate the inspector's audit and improve the outcome.

A Few Comments About Audits

It is not in the scope of this book to go into FDA audits in detail, but we can share some of the wisdom gained since PBRC opened in 1993. Our experience suggests that inspectors are particularly interested in the correspondence

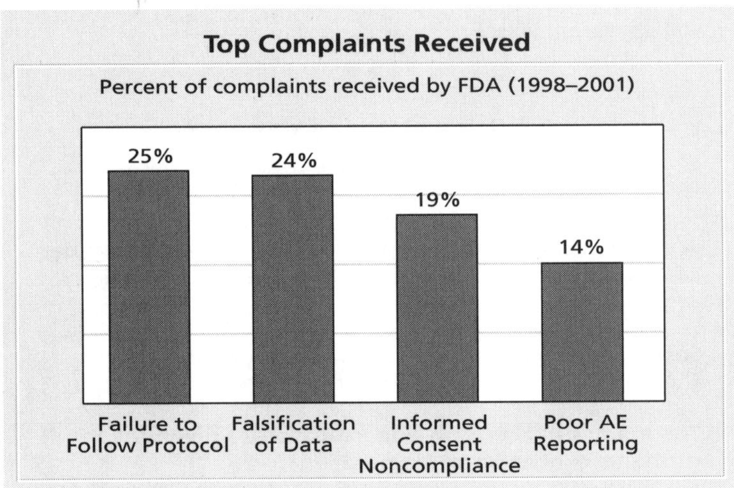

Figure 2 Source: FDA Division of Safety Inspection, CenterWatch Analyses

section of the regulatory binder because any problems with studies become obvious in this section. Any communications with the IRB or sponsors addressing problems about the study are in this section.

Within the first five minutes of visiting your site, the FDA inspector usually develops a good sense as to whether there is a problem. If staff act nervous and worried, the inspector will suspect that they have reason to be and will probably be justified in that suspicion. If, however, the clinical staff is secure about the quality of the data, has been following the site's SOPs and has properly maintained the regulatory binder, this will also be obvious to the inspector. The investigator and sub-investigator should be present for the inspection.

The auditor's job is to ensure that regulations designed to protect the rights and safety of human subjects are being followed along with aspects of good clinical practice (GCP) leading to ethical development of investigational compounds and devices. With this in mind, it is best to go through the audit in the spirit in which it is intended.

Helpful Hints to Improve Site Performance and Outcome of Audits
A visiting CRO shared valuable information regarding audit preparation. Not only is it necessary to lock controlled substances in a drug room, placed in a locked safe or locked cabinet, but it is also necessary to have the safe or drug cabinet bolted to the floor or wall.
Failure to follow drug storage protocol or maintain drug accountability logs warrants an automatic Form 483.
It is important to maintain equipment maintenance logs. It is a good idea to assign someone on the administrative staff to check the thermometers each day and keep the logs current. Multiple 483s have been filed against sites that did not have maintenance logs for various pieces of equipment.

Table 8

On the final day of the FDA audit, the inspector will conduct an exit interview. During this interview, the FDA inspector will discuss findings. For this reason, it is helpful if the site's top management can sit in at this meeting. It is preferable to have the CEO, DCO, principal investigator and QA director present. The QA director should take notes during this meeting. Our experience at PBRC suggests that you will have to ask the inspector if these members of the management team can attend. Sometimes, the inspector will not permit all of these people to be present, allowing only the primary investigator and the QA director.

If warranted, the inspector will issue a written Form FDA-483, an "inspectional observations" form that is used to notify the site's top management of significant conditions relating to products or processes observed during the inspection.

Following the inspection, the FDA generally issues one of three types of letters to the investigator:[ix]

1. A notice that no significant deviations from the regulations were observed. This letter does not require any response. (No action indicated, NAI.)

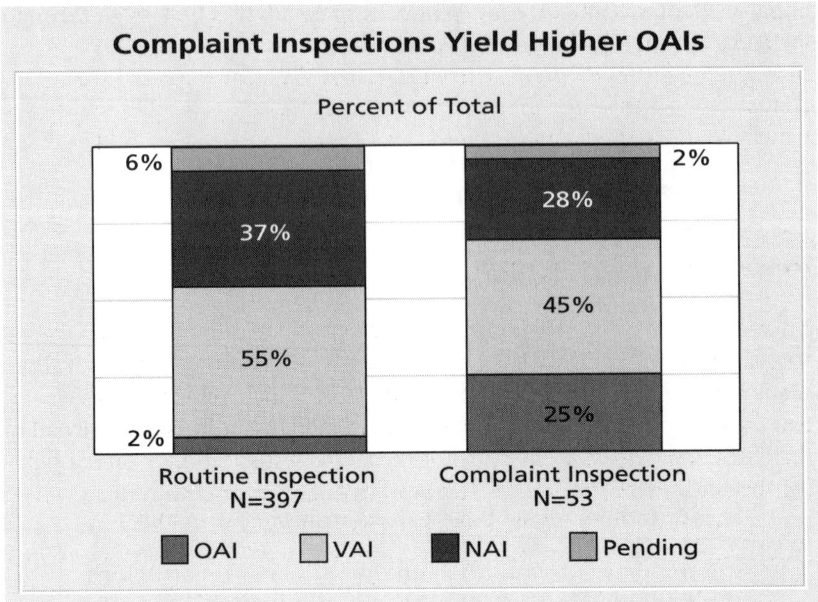

Figure 3

Source: CenterWatch, FDA 2001

2. An informational letter identifying deviations from regulations and good investigational practice. This letter may or may not require a response from the clinical investigator. If a response is requested, the letter will describe what is necessary for follow-up. (Voluntary action indicated, VAI.)

3. A Warning Letter identifying serious deviations from regulations requiring prompt correction by the clinical investigator. The letter will provide the name of a contact person for questions. In these cases, the FDA may inform both the study sponsor and the IRB of the deficiencies. The Agency may also inform the sponsor if the investigator's procedural deficiencies indicate ineffective monitoring by the sponsor. In addition to issuing these letters, the FDA may take other courses of action, such as regulatory and/or administrative sanctions. (Official action indicated, OAI.)

The quality assurance and regulatory affairs departments can seek to limit deficiencies that auditors may find by paying particular attention to the most commonly found deficiencies in FDA audits. Results of FDA site audits in 2000 showed that protocol non-compliance was the most frequently cited deficiency, followed by record-keeping deficiencies, such as source documentation not matching case report forms (Figure 3). It is worth remembering that inspectors may find fault with even the most perfectly completed CRFs. For example, if a physician has hurriedly signed his or her name to acknowledge receipt of a laboratory value, resulting in a signature looking slightly different than it did on all the other report forms, it could be construed as a possible forgery, even though it isn't. When the quality assurance and regulatory affairs departments are preparing for the audit, they should review the patient charts and regulatory binder with the critical eye of an FDA auditor.

Inspections by Sponsors

An audit by the sponsor tends to occur when the site is involved in a pivotal trial, the sponsor and/or CRO believes there is a problem at the site or if the site is a high enroller. The sponsor inspection, which generally lasts one or two days, tends to be more complete than the FDA audit, as generally all of the CRFs are reviewed. The spirit of the sponsor inspection is one of helping the site. Indeed, what a site learns from the sponsor inspection can help it prepare for an FDA audit. Also, a positive inspection can help the site to grow because at least that sponsor and the affiliated CRO will be aware that the site is functioning ethically and effectively and is a good candidate for future work.

In Review

This chapter has highlighted necessary ingredients for growing a site into a larger, highly professional operation. They include the addition of a Director of Clinical Operations (DCO), development of departments of quality assurance and regulatory affairs, the setting up and implementation of standard operating procedures (SOPs) and hiring of a data manager. The goal is for the staff to work together to improve the quality of clinical trials at the site, leading to greater patient safety and improved outcomes of visits from monitors and visits from auditors from the Food and Drug Administration and from sponsors.

The site needs all of these staff positions to facilitate the dividing up of the many pieces of the study conduct pie into manageable bites. For example, developing and maintaining SOPs is too important a task to relegate to someone who is already consumed with the details of study conduct. The same holds true for the regulatory binder. The binder must be constantly maintained, and this can only be accomplished by a staff member dedicated to this purpose. Using this approach, the site will grow in an organized, regulatory-compliant manner.

References

i "The Value of Site-Based Quality Assurance Systems for Clinical Testing Sites," *The Monitor*, R.A. Koshore Nadkarni, Shelley Antel, and Karen Sargent, Winter 2000, Vol. 14, Issue 4, p. 29.

ii Definition of Quality Assurance, *http://praxiom.com*, accessed May 1, 2001.

iii "Guidance for Industry Good Clinical Practice: Consolidated Guidance," Center for Drug Evaluation and Research, April 1996, p. 1.

iv "The Value of Site-Based Quality Assurance Systems for Clinical Testing Sites," *The Monitor*, R.A. Koshore Nadkarni, Shelley Antel, and Karen Sargent, Winter 2000, Vol. 14, Issue 4, p. 30.

v Ibid., *The Monitor*, p. 30.

vi *http://www.fda.gov/oc/ohrt/irbs/operations.html#inspections*, accessed May 10, 2001.

vii Ibid., accessed May 10, 2001.

viii *http://www.fda.gov/cder/present/dia-62000/woolen1/tsld032.htm*, accessed May 10, 2001.

ix *http://www.fda.gov/oc/ohrt/irbs/operations.html#inspections*, accessed May 10, 2001.

CHAPTER 5

Business Development

- A Multi-Faceted Approach Is Best
- Develop a Professional Brochure and Matching Materials
- Send Materials to the Site Selector
- Make Use of Print- and Web-Based Resources
- Your Own Web Site
- Form Business Relationships
- Monitors
- Other Ways to Establish Good Business Relationships
- Attend Professional Meetings
- Presentations at Professional Meetings
- To Exhibit or Not to Exhibit
- Work Those Investigator Meetings
- Attend End-of-Study Meetings
- In Review

Over the years, our marketing staff has expanded to three full-time professionals, and our marketing budget has grown to the point that it now represents approximately 10% of gross revenues. Due largely to their efforts and our understanding of the importance of continually promoting our site, we now conduct several dozen studies simultaneously across our five sites in South Florida. Part of their job includes keeping an eye on the changing trends in the industry as certain therapeutic areas, and the associated clinical trials, wax and wane in popularity. According to the Pharmaceutical Research and Manufacturers of America (PhRMA), the top six areas of clinical research based on R&D dollars are:[i]

- Cancers
- CNS and Sense Organs
- Neoplasms, Endocrine and Metabolism
- Cardiovascular Disease
- Infective and Parasitic Diseases
- Digestion and Genito-Urinary System
- Respiratory System
- Dermatology

This chapter is designed as an overview of practical and effective methods of promoting the ongoing development of business at the investigative site.

A Multi-Faceted Approach Is Best

As anxious as you are to make contacts with sponsors and CROs, they are equally so. They need to place studies in a timely fashion at qualified sites with experienced investigators. Successful growth strategies require a multi-faceted approach and budget commitment. Making a few phone calls won't do it, nor will just mailing out a few or even hundreds of brochures when research indicates direct mail generally yields a 0.5% to 1% response or sales rate. If you mail 200 brochures with a well-crafted cover letter, you can expect a response from one or two.[ii] You may get lucky and get a few trials, but typically the level of response is insufficient to stay in business or to cover print costs.

A busy, successful plastic surgeon once said, "It's not what you do in your practice, it's everything that you do." This philosophy applies to business development for the investigative site. More than one step has to be taken and the effort must be coupled with dollars earmarked for marketing purposes. A study of 103 investigative sites revealed that on average, 5% of gross revenues are spent on site marketing initiatives.[iii]

Besides making a plan and funding it, building relationships within the clinical trials community is also key to a site's success. Clinical research is very much a relationships business, so all interactions with clinical partners, i.e., sponsors, CROs, SMOs, independents sites, should be oriented toward building lasting relationships and friendships.

Some site promotion tactics include:*

- Development of a high-quality brochure and folder
- Development of a well-written cover letter on company letterhead
- Development of an accurate list of sponsors and CROs with current names and addresses
- Use of industry publications

* The subject of paid advertising is noticeably absent from this list. Although the placement of advertisement in industry journals will create awareness of your site, it is generally more expensive and yields fewer results than other methods listed here.

- Use of Internet resources
- Development of a web site
- Development of close relationships with clinical partners, i.e., sponsors, monitors, CROs, other sites
- Joining industry-related associations and committees of interest
- Attendance at industry trade shows
- Presenting at industry trade shows
- Networking at investigator meetings
- Attendance at end-of-study meetings
- Presenting to sponsors or CROs at their home offices

Develop a Professional Brochure, Matching Materials

Having the flashiest brochure in town doesn't guarantee a quality operation or necessarily translate into lots of business, but it does suggest that your site is serious about the clinical trials business. And it does attract attention. Projecting a highly professional image is the first step in promoting an investigative site. This starts with investing in the design and printing of a professional brochure and folder that touts a company logo. This creates an immediately recognizable identity for your company. The brochure and folder should be designed either by an advertising or graphics professional unless you or someone on your staff is creative and familiar with the various types of graphic design software. Matching letterhead and business cards complete the package.

The brochure is your advertising piece. It needs to capture the essence and uniqueness of your site by promoting past achievements and current capabilities. It might promote a specialty in oncology trials or the fact that the site has an experienced, bilingual staff. Access to thought leaders in specific, "hot" therapeutic areas is also worth mentioning. Finally, getting testimonials from sponsors or CROs you have worked with is eye-catching and establishes credibility. A few catch phrases might be, "Best site we ever worked with," "Produces high-quality data," "Professional, well-trained staff," "Fast turnaround on regulatory documents, budgets and contracts" or "Always reaches or exceeds our enrollment targets."

When soliciting business, we mail folders containing our site brochure and a cover letter targeted to the prospective client. We use the cover letter to present information about our track record for enrollment on related studies, always being mindful to maintain confidentiality. For example, if we are soliciting business for a COPD trial, we might mention that in a previous COPD trial, we enrolled thirty patients, 200% above the ten for which we originally contracted. We may cite additional trials in related areas for which we over-enrolled in an expedient manner.[ii] In addition, we enclose curriculum vitae (CVs) of appropriate investigators. But, we are careful not to overemphasize the overenrolling of studies as this could raise a red flag about the possible use of coercive techniques.

Send Materials to the Site Selector

The best brochure, cover letter and folder are wasted if they are sent to the wrong people. In an industry where people are constantly being reshuffled, it is important to find out the names, job titles and addresses of site selectors before undertaking a mailing. In a 2001 CenterWatch survey of forty-five sponsors, CROs, SMOs and independent sites, 73% of respondents reported that company turnover was either very significant or somewhat significant. The same study revealed that project managers average a four-year tenure, and monitors, just three years.[iv]

While turnover contributes to problems in finding the right site selector, so does the fact that each sponsor handles site selection differently. Site selection responsibility may rest with the project manager at one sponsor, the medical director at another and with the site selector at a third. Sometimes, the CRO handles site selection.

An experienced site might ask visiting monitors for the names of current site selectors in various therapeutic areas. Some monitors will know of a few site selectors, others will not. A new site still trying to procure its first few studies will not have the luxury of having visiting monitors to quiz. They will have to be persistent, meaning that they will have to call, fax and/or email the sponsors to try to gather this information. Because site selectors travel frequently, they are often unavailable for telephone calls, but may respond to e-mail. Being persistent, without being annoying, will eventually pay off.

Example 1 – Finding the Site Selector

Several years ago, I saw a story on CNN about a then upcoming trial for an AIDS vaccine. Subsequently, I read about the same trial. I was impressed with the possibilities for the vaccine and felt a strong personal commitment to this type of research. I liked the idea of being able to tell my grandchildren that I had participated in this important work.

After expressing my keen interest to the marketing department, our marketing director went in relentless pursuit of the site selector for this study. He called the sponsor, CNN and the publication where I had seen the article. After several weeks, he found the site selector.

Not only did PBRC end up as a selected site, it was the only independent site in this multi-center trial. All the others were either health clinics or academic medical centers. We were proud to participate in this trial and were proud of the marketing department for having accomplished this feat.

Make Use of Print- and Web-Based Resources

Numerous print and web-based publications are designed to help sites identify clinical trials opportunities as well as promote themselves, two factors critical to continued success. At PBRC, we consider these print and electronic publications as integral to our business development plan because we have secured many research grants as a direct result of participating in or using these resources.

In the print realm, *Clinical Investigator News*, published monthly by CTB International, provides information on which compounds are being targeted for which indications, where they are being researched, where they stand in the clinical trials pipeline and names of contacts who handle clinical research grants. Within each medical specialty, items are organized by stage of development, starting with pre-clinical and advancing through phases I, II, III and IV. Subscription information is available either by calling 973-379-7749 or by logging on to *www.ctbintl.com.*

PharmaBusiness, a print publication appearing seven times annually, offers an international view on a variety of topics, including news and marketing issues specific to the clinical research sector. Its summer issue, "What's in the Pipeline" is particularly useful as it reviews more than 5,000 products that are moving through the clinical development pipeline, from pre-clinical to those that are awaiting FDA approval. "What's in the Pipeline" is also available on CD-ROM as a searchable database and is arranged by therapeutic area, status, dosage form, developer, marketer, indications and more. In January 2002, online database capability is being launched as part of a suite of products known as eKnowledgeBase. Print subscription information is available at *www.pharmalive.com/pharma_month/flash/3003.asp* and information on the electronic database products can be found at *www.pharmalive.com.datase_products/4000_f.asp*.

CenterWatch, the publisher of this book, and a publishing and information service for the clinical trials industry, has extensive print and Internet-based resources. The monthly print newsletter, *CenterWatch*, contains sections entitled "Grant Opportunities" and "TrialWatch." The Grant Opportunities feature selects different therapeutic areas each month and lists investigational products by phase and sponsor. TrialWatch provides a list of companies that have confirmed that they are seeking investigators for therapeutic-specific studies about to begin. Contact names and telephone numbers are included in both sections. Subscription information is available at 800-765-9647 or at *www.centerwatch.com/bookstore/pubs_profs_cwnews.html.*

The CenterWatch web site, *www.centerwatch.com*, presents patients and industry with easy-to-use information designed to:

- Help patients find local industry- and government-sponsored clinical trials in therapeutic areas of interest

- Help sponsors and CROs locate investigative sites with experience in specific therapeutic areas by listing profiles of hundreds of clinical research centers
- Help investigative sites gain access to patients by listing currently enrolling trials and contact information

CenterWatch reports that its Web site has more than 500,000 visitors monthly.

The *Clinical Investigators Directory*, an annual publication of Research Investigator's Source, Inc. provides an extensive listing of individual investigators, investigative sites, site management organizations (SMOs), contract research organizations (CROs) and laboratories. Information on types of studies conducted by sites and investigators, academic affiliations of the investigators, years in the business and contact information are included. Listings are cross-referenced by specialty, geographic location and therapeutic areas.

The directory is available in print and web-based formats. Sponsors seeking investigators for clinical trials have free access to the online directory and can order a complimentary hard copy by ordering from the web address given below. Investigative sites and clinical investigators seeking to be listed in the print and online directories should contact the publisher at 763-591-7790 or *www.clinicalinvestigators.com.*

Your Own Web Site

An investigative site may opt to build its own web site for promotional purposes. Although sponsors and CROs seeking investigators are likely to use established resources such as *www.centerwatch.com* or *Clinical Investigators Directory*, they may also scan sites to pick up additional or more updated information. Prospective patients who may be unfamiliar with industry resources may know of local clinical research centers through local patient recruitment advertisements and may search the web using of the names of those local centers. Many investigative sites use their web sites to list currently enrolling and upcoming trials. They generally enable prospective subjects to enter names, addresses, telephone numbers and email addresses for future contact.

Probably the best way to design a web site is to scan several that are already online to get a sense of their user-friendliness and how they are organized. On the most basic level, a site needs to post its mission statement, its therapeutic specialties, location with directions and contact information. It may also want to have one route for patients and another for industry. Tables 1 and 2 list patient-oriented and industry-oriented topics, respectively, that may appear on a web site.

Web sites are part of the overall marketing strategy, the goal being to entice the site selector to call for further information. Similarly, information appearing on the web site may pique the interest of prospective patients, but usually, it is only through a telephone conversation with a well-trained patient recruiter that the patient will decide to be screened. Despite the advances of technology, people still want to deal with human beings. It is the basis of all business.

Patient-Oriented Topics on Your Web Site
Explanation of clinical research trials
Explanation of informed consent
General information about your site
Listings of currently enrolling and soon-to-be-enrolling studies
Space for prospective subjects to submit questions and contact information

Table 1

Industry-Oriented Topics on Your Web Site
Capabilities in various therapeutic areas
Trial experience
Size of the site
A statement about the site's focus on quality
Profile of Research Team principal investigators
Equipment
Contact information

Table 2

Form Business Relationships

In the clinical trials industry, as in nearly all others, forming business relationships with prospective clients and nourishing relationships with existing clients are fundamental to making a business flourish. The old saw, "People like to do business with people they like," certainly holds true in this sector. Sites that have been successful with past studies and have developed a good rapport with site selectors and other clinical team members can expect to enjoy repeat business from those same CROs and sponsors. This is critical to site survival and growth because all dollars for industry-sponsored trials flow from the sponsors. For this reason, a key element in a multi-faceted business development strategy calls for meeting as many people in the industry as possible, and treating them in the same respectful manner in which you expect to be treated. While reaching enrollment targets in a timely fashion and producing clean, reliable data will always be the hallmarks of a quality site, a site will have a difficult time demonstrating its quality until a sponsor or CRO is convinced to select it. This starts with building a relationship, and this takes planning and perseverance.

Many sponsors and CROs are large, multi-national corporations, in which people in one department often do not know people in another. Consequently, if a site has performed well in a diabetes trial, that in no way suggests that the site will have a better than average chance of securing a migraine trial from that same sponsor or CRO.

To complicate matters further, employees of the sponsors and CROs move around, either within the same company or to a new company. While job changers may bring their file of past contacts with them to their new employer, this does not guarantee that the person will have the same or even similar responsibilities for site selection, and his or her old job may be filled by someone you don't know or someone who has no knowledge of your site.

Monitors

Sites can stay on top of this frequent uprooting of established contacts, in part. Staying in touch with other sites, or asking visiting monitors "What's new?" will help the site tap into news circulating in the industry. Monitors, or clinical research associates (CRAs), are the representatives of the sponsor or CRO visiting your site to review that protocol is being adhered to and the data are being properly collected, recorded and forwarded. Monitors often maintain a heavy travel schedule and may not always receive warm receptions at the sites they visit. Some sites may consider the monitor visit an intrusion into their busy day.

This line of thinking is definitely misguided. In the spirit of trying to build positive relationships that will help the site attract new business, it is always best to treat monitors with respect and enable them to perform their work in a welcoming atmosphere.

At PBRC, we provide monitors with a handout that lists nearby places to eat and shop, as well as popular tourist sites. Our monitor workroom is equipped with coffee and a refrigerator filled with snacks and drinks to make their visits more comfortable. We try to make our site more of a destination, rather than just another site to pore over case report forms. In addition, we value their input by asking them to complete a monitor's evaluation form of our site and of our coordinators. We solicit comments as to how we can improve our site and make it more user-friendly to monitors.

We believe this approach helps establish the kind of relationship to enable us to ask visiting monitors about other trials the sponsor has under way or is planning. If the monitor is self-employed, we ask about current and upcoming trials from multiple sponsors. We also ask if he or she can provide contact names, particularly those of site selectors. Monitors with good, long-term relationships often go out of their way to provide information about upcoming studies. Over the years, this approach has resulted in PBRC learning about various trials we eventually secured.

Other Ways to Establish Good Business Relationships

Another tactic is to become active in trade associations such as the Drug Information Association (DIA), the American Academy of Pharmaceutical Physicians (AAPP), the Association of Clinical Research Professionals (ACRP), and the Society of Clinical Research Associates (SoCRA).

Other methods for establishing good business relationships are:

- Attend professional meetings
- Attend investigator meetings
- Attend end-of-study meetings

Some of the larger CROs maintain premier-site or preferred-site programs. The criteria for acceptance vary from company to company, but as the titles suggest, these programs enable participating sites to have business steered to them first before going outside of the preferred network. The designated sites are often high quality and high performing, and those selected often develop a good working relationship, facilitating the exchange of leads. Contact various CROs to learn which ones maintain these programs.

Attend Professional Meetings

Clinical investigators are generally very busy people, but the successful ones know the value of attending at least a few local, regional or national meetings each year. Some of the more visible national associations are profiled here.

The largest gathering in the pharmaceutical industry is the annual North American meeting of the Drug Information Association (DIA). Each year, more than 10,000 representatives of academia, contract service organizations, regulatory affairs, investigative sites, pharmaceutical, biotechnology and medical device manufacturers come together for this mega-meeting. Because of the sheer size of the event, it can be challenging to exchange meaningful dialogue with prospective clients, but it can provide young sites with a sense of the scope and dimension of the clinical trials industry.

Visiting the exhibit booths of sponsors and CROs gives opportunities for attendees to meet and speak with people who are equally anxious to meet and speak with them. This interaction will mark the first step in building your network of relationships. Bring lots of business cards and site brochures.

The receptions are excellent for networking. They offer a chance to meet site selectors in an informal setting. For this reason, it is wise to target six or seven receptions in one evening. Because it is unlikely that one person could attend so many events in one night, it might be a good idea to bring a few of your staff members so they can divide up the various receptions. Visit *http://events.diahome.org/search.asp* for information on the annual DIA meeting and the numerous DIA workshops held throughout the year.

DIA also hosts an annual European meeting which is much smaller and is focused on the specific needs of its European members. Although this

Some Committees of the American Academy of Pharmaceutical Physicians

Committees
AMA Relations
Annual Meeting
Education Committee
Ethics Committee
Fellowship Committee
International Relations Committee
Public Affairs Committee
Seminars Committee
Strategic Planning Committee

Table 3 Source: www.aapp.org

meeting is a more manageable size, thereby facilitating direct interaction with sponsors and CROs, it will probably be less beneficial for business development purposes than its North American counterpart.

The American Academy of Pharmaceutical Physicians (AAPP) hosts an annual meeting. This gathering is worthwhile because its small size, about 200 attendees, facilitates interacting and mingling with upper level management and medical directors from sponsors and CROs who also attend. This is an invaluable chance to spend one-on-one time with people who are positioned to offer research grants or can steer you toward individuals at their organizations with this authority.

AAPP targets physicians who devote a substantial portion of their time to basic and clinical research, clinical trial design and outcomes research. The organization also has various committees (Table 3) which enable members to meet and work with other physicians from all aspects of the clinical trials industry. Membership is open to physicians (MDs, DOs, MBBSs) in good standing. For further information, call 919-355-1000 or visit *www.aapp.org*.

The Association of Clinical Research Professionals (ACRP) and the Society of Clinical Research Associates (SoCRA) both sponsor annual meetings. Although these meetings are geared more toward monitors and study coordinators, a number of investigators do attend. Many of the sessions offer the latest information on trends in clinical research from the site's perspective. There are numerous exhibitors and receptions that provide networking opportunities. The ACRP meeting averages 3,000 attendees. Information is available at 202-737-8100 or *www.acrpnet.org*. SoCRA's annual meeting has an attendance of some 500 to 600. This association can be reached at 215-345-7749 or *www.socra.org*. Both organizations offer committees and regional chapters.

It is worth mentioning that annual meetings can be used for more than networking opportunities between your site and sponsors and CROs. It is also important to network with other sites to solidify working relationships, a tactic that incurs no additional marketing costs. These sites should be viewed as a source of lead and information sharing, and not as a source of competition because, generally, they are from other regions of the country. Taking the time to plan get-togethers with other sites is usually necessary at annual meetings because otherwise, they won't happen.

Presentations at Professional Meetings

Annual meetings bring together hundreds, and in some cases, thousands of people. With this many individuals in attendance, each with a different agenda, gaining visibility for your site takes definite planning. We discussed the value of touring the exhibit booths and visiting at least some of the receptions. Another strategy is to give a presentation or prepare a poster board. While both require a great deal of preparation, they do focus a bit of undivided attention onto your site. I had the experience of giving a few presentations at a large annual meeting only to have a sponsor practically chase me down the hall after one of them to offer a large study to PBRC. As of this writing, the study has been ongoing for the past four years, and it remains one of our more successful ventures in terms of patient enrollment and retention.

Information about the presentations and poster sessions can serve as a source of free advertising for your site as it generally appears in direct mailings about the conference, their print publications and is usually posted on the organizations' web sites prior to the meeting. It often remains there for a very long time, usually at least one year, sometimes longer. Benefits of these presentations can be further extended. A summary of your presentation or poster board can be attached to a letter of solicitation to potential clients, or to a regular "Dear Contact" letter to existing clients. The posters can be framed and placed in the meeting room at your site so that they are visible to all visiting sponsors, CROs and monitors.

To Exhibit or Not to Exhibit

When PBRC was a young site, we thought it was important to have an exhibit booth at the DIA and ACRP annual meetings. We spent upwards of $20,000 to have a good-looking, professional, easily portable booth made. While we believe that a site planning to exhibit is best represented by a professional-looking booth, we also believe that a site's money might be better spent circulating among the other exhibit booths and attending meetings and receptions. A booth has to have a representative from your site in it at all times, meaning that "circulation time" is reduced and your site has to send enough people to the meeting to cover all the exhibit hours.

There is another pitfall to bringing lots of staff to a meeting for the purposes of having someone in the booth continuously—your study coordinators may be amazed at how large the industry is and by the many job opportunities for monitors. The ACRP meeting, in particular, has a job fair, and all of our study coordinators must have scoped it out. Within six months of their attending their first ACRP conference, all of them quit PBRC to enter monitor training programs with sponsors. These coordinators had been inexperienced when we hired them, so we had trained them ourselves.

This experience taught us two invaluable lessons. We learned to think twice about whom we take to meetings, but more importantly, it forced us to re-evaluate whom we hire as study coordinators. As discussed in the chapter "Keeping Your Study Coordinator," we now seek experienced coordinators who make patient contact a priority, something that is lacking in a monitor's job. Those seeking time flexibility to balance family and work responsibilities and express little interest in the inordinate amount of travel that is expected of many monitors are less likely to be wooed by openings posted at meetings for good-paying monitor positions. On the positive side, it is possible to use the job fair to your advantage. You can advertise openings at your center, and perhaps interview several well-qualified candidates.

Work Those Investigator Meetings

While the purpose of an investigator meeting is to learn about the protocol, they provide some of the best networking opportunities. The fact that your site was selected for the study means that it met some established criteria. Perhaps these sponsors and CROs will be in a position to select or recommend your site for future studies. There are several steps you can take to increase the likelihood of that happening (Table 4).

First, project a professional image at all meetings. Because you never get a second chance to make a first impression, it is important to dress professionally. Many times, I have attended investigator meetings where some of the principal investigators showed up in jogging suits or torn jeans. Coordinators sometimes look disheveled. While statistics probably do not exist linking mode of dress at investigator meetings to rate of securing new studies, it is only common sense that sponsors and CROs will be drawn to individuals who have enough respect to appear professional and interested.

It is a good idea to attend the reception the night before, and be on time. Many investigators fail to show up for the reception, attending only the meeting on the following day. I have found that if you arrive five or ten minutes early for the reception, the only people in the room are usually those from the sponsor and the CRO. This is a golden opportunity to have a few moments of their undivided attention. Not only will this demonstrate your enthusiasm for the project, it will enable you to ask about future projects. I always exchange business cards at these receptions. When I return from the meeting, our marketing department uses the collected business cards to send follow-up letters to each individual, attaching background information about PBRC. We also add their email addresses to our electronic address book and use them to send periodic emails about activities of interest at our site.

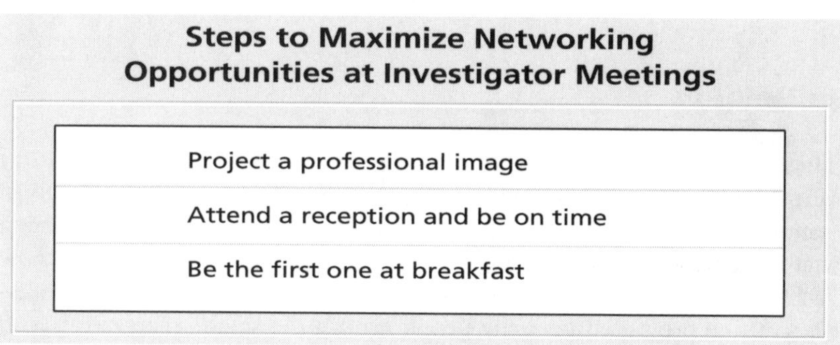

Steps to Maximize Networking Opportunities at Investigator Meetings
Project a professional image
Attend a reception and be on time
Be the first one at breakfast

Table 4

Another good pointer is be first at breakfast because the people from the sponsor and CRO and key speakers show up early. Few attendees take advantage of this opportunity, so typically there are plenty of seats available at these tables. I often eat breakfast with them and try to form some type of business relationship. In this type of intimate setting, it is easy to start an informal conversation.

Attend End-of-Study Meetings

PBRC was in business for several years before I recognized the importance of end-of-study meetings. Before I attended my first one, I tended to ignore them under the guise that I was "too busy." These meetings are held for several reasons, but they are usually held when the trial has been very successful and/or the sponsor wants to share with the investigators what it considers to be significant results.

I attended my first end-of-study meeting in San Francisco following the completion of a successful trial for a new migraine compound. We were wined and dined and housed in one of the best hotels in the city. The sponsor took us on a tour of San Francisco harbor after bestowing us with an exquisite dinner and small gifts to show its appreciation for our efforts. Barely 15% of the investigators showed up for this meeting. Interestingly, the investigators who did come were all seasoned principal investigators from well-known sites.

This meeting still ranks as one of my most productive networking experiences. I made contacts with top-flight sites from across the country that were in a position to share leads. I was fortunate to meet several of the sponsor's marketing staff, the project manager and a few others involved in running the trial. Through this fun and informal setting, I established contacts that have contributed to our site's business development to this day.

Since that time, I make it a point to attend all the end-of-study meetings, if possible. They can offer a helpful boost to business development efforts. This is one of the little known pearls in the industry.

In Review

There is no one right way to develop business for your site. In an industry where people come and go, and where therapeutic areas come and go in popularity, it is important to use a multitude of approaches. Recognizing that sponsors employ thousands of people means that many do not know each other, so the value that your site can bring to the clinical trials process needs to be promoted to many people within the same organization, and often, more than once. Sending letters and brochures to the right decision makers, following up with one or more telephone calls and e-mails, arranging to meet at industry get-togethers and becoming active in industry associations are all part of the process of establishing valuable relationships in the clinical trials industry. The key is to be proactive.

PBRC has grown to the point that it now has three full-time staff members dedicated to business development activities. They are a very organized and aggressive group yet despite their best efforts, we are constantly amazed at the number of industry representatives we uncover who are unaware of our site's existence. Certainly with nine years experience and five locations, we are one of the more established independent sites, but the very fact that many in the industry do not know we exist highlights the critical importance of constantly marketing the site. The industry is always in flux, so your site needs the foundation of established relationships to keep informed of industry trends and changes; otherwise it will be left behind.

References

i Pharmaceutical Research and Manufacturers of America (PhRMA), *www.PhRMA.org/publications/publications/profile01/chapter2.phtml#allocation*, accessed October 9, 2001.

ii Small Business Administration, *http://www.onlinewbc.org/docs/market/mk_dirmail.html.*

iii "Sites Prosper...but Financial Health Threatened," *CenterWatch*, Vol. 7, Issue 1, January 2000, Lisa Henderson, Lisa Wilder, p. 11.

iv "Evolving Employment Trends in the Clinical Trials Industry," DIA Annual Meeting 2001, Joan A. Kroll, CenterWatch; Marianne Considine, Advanced Clinical Services.

CHAPTER 6

Partnering with Investigators and Other Important Agreements

- How to Find a Good Fit Before Partnering
- Successful Contracting with Investigators
- Coordinators: Make It a Win/Win
- Contracting with Other Sites
- Site Indemnification
- In Review

As your site expands, you will invariably need to sign written contracts with various clinical partners. Contracts play an important role in the clinical trials industry because they outline the formal agreements between sites and investigators; sites and other sites; sites and sponsors; and sites and CROs. The purpose of each contract is to enhance or facilitate clinical research at your site. The best contracts are concise and about three or four pages in length. Agreements that are extremely difficult to understand and read usually do not hold up well.

A contract is a legally binding promise between parties to perform specific tasks in exchange for consideration. A letter of agreement can also be used. It is generally less formal and its purpose may be to avoid the legal consequences of a contract. Negotiating favorable contracts and letters of agreement can be time-consuming, but they are necessary business tools for growth. The contracts included in this chapter are examples used to present various concepts. They are not intended for use.

We advise you to consult an attorney to protect your interests when engaging in any contracting. A health care attorney who has experience dealing with physicians would be the ideal choice. If you are unable to find a health care attorney, another good choice would be a business attorney. Any type of agreement between physicians should be straightforward.

Ultimately, physicians with integrity will not break a contract, and those who are less ethical will not abide by any contract you have them sign. PBRC has had physicians sign non-compete agreements with us for a minimum period of a year. A week or two later these same physicians have gone out and started up their own studies, in spite of the contract. They had used us as a way to educate themselves about how to do clinical trials. At this point, we had a business decision to make—whether to take them to court and hold them to the contract or just let them go. We felt there was nothing to gain by taking these physicians to court. It's a difficult business and not as easy as it seemed for them to survive. Most of these physicians who have broken their contract have lost a lot of money, and their sites have only survived a year or so. They had to stop doing trials because of the financial and operating burdens and their failure to secure additional business. They lost out, but so did we. The best first step to partnering with anyone is to pick the right partner.

How to Find a Good Fit Before Partnering

The best method for growing your investigative site is by expanding your capabilities into a variety of therapeutic areas. Clinical research grants are spread over numerous specialties, and sites positioned to perform many types of quality studies will have greater access to those study dollars. Gearing up for expanded offerings means signing contracts with local area specialists who have the time and inclination to conduct clinical research. It is a good idea to have signed contracts in place with specialists before bidding on studies in those therapeutic areas.

Finding those physicians can be a challenge because a good physician is not necessarily a good clinical investigator. We have developed specific indicators that provide clues as to whether a particular physician will be a cooperative and productive investigator. When we first approach a physician to be a potential investigator, we follow up initial discussions by sending a confidentiality agreement. If he or she signs it and returns it promptly, that is a good sign. Just this simple test eliminates approximately 80% to 90% of the physicians we approach.

We also closely monitor how quickly they provide information we request about their patient databases and the usefulness of those databases. For example, is the database searchable by "number of rheumatoid arthritis and osteoarthritis patients seen per month and per week" or is it broken down only by "arthritis"? Can the database be searched by "patients with primary hypertension" as well as by "hypertensive patients who also have cardiac disease"? If not, does the doctor have the software to pull up this information by International Classification of Disease (ICD-9) codes? Additional indicators appear in Table 1.

When physicians approach us about becoming clinical investigators, we generally look for physicians who are willing to be trained in how to conduct clinical research in accordance with good clinical practice (GCP). Money is a good short-term motivator, but long-term, the physician needs to be motivated in things other than money such as research and being associated with cutting-edge findings. The best candidate is a physician who is not fitting research in between many other interests and commitments and who can make research his or her prime focus.

Indicators That a Physician Is Likely to be a Good Clinical Investigator
Signs confidentiality statement and returns it in a timely fashion
Forwards license and DEA certificate in a timely fashion
Willing to sign restrictive covenant
Fills out questionnaire about patient population and returns it promptly
Has patients who might qualify for studies
Reads prospective protocol
Returns calls promptly
Willing to provide beeper number, home number and cell phone number
Is a physician you would have treat you or your family

Table 1

Training physicians associated with your site is critical because untrained or undertrained investigators may be unaware of the complexities and ramifications involved in violating the protocol, improperly obtaining informed consent or not disclosing potential financial conflicts of interest. A recent article in *The Monitor*, the publication of the Association of Clinical Research Professionals (ACRP), reports results of a membership survey in which 56% of 2040 respondents ranked the need to train investigators as the most important area of training.[i] To address this need, ACRP launched a three-day pilot course in December 2000 entitled, "Good Clinical Practices for Investigators," which is a training program followed by two years of peer-support and mentoring. The course was developed in response to ACRP survey results, sponsor input and to the numerous government initiatives through the Department of Health and Human Services (HHS) aimed at raising the investigators' knowledge of proper trial conduct.[ii]

Some investigators need to improve their level of protocol compliance. In 2000, the Center for Drug Evaluation and Research (CDER) a division of the Food and Drug Administration, reported that the most frequently cited deficiency in 305 FDA audits conducted that year was protocol noncompliance by the investigator. This accounted for 35% of all deficiencies identified (Figure 1). Our site has had direct experience with this problem.

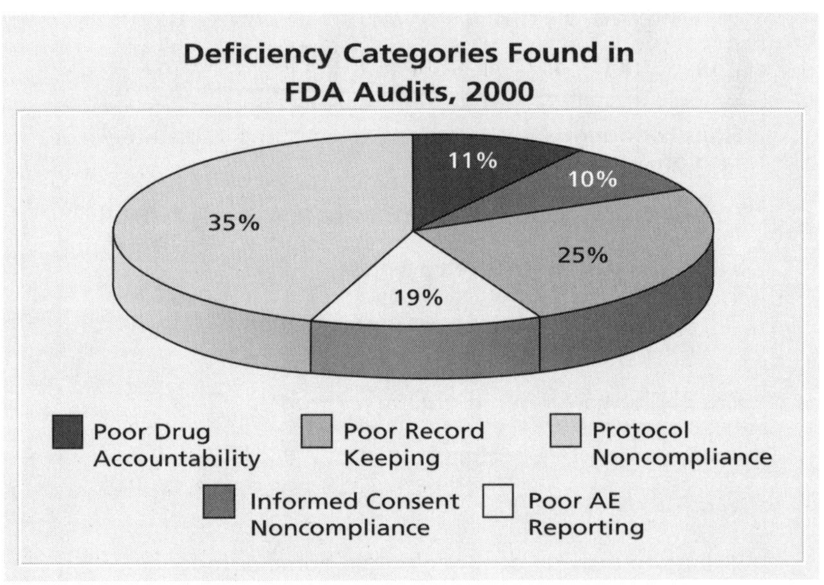

Figure 1 Source: FDA Division of Safety Inspection, CenterWatch Analyses 2000

Example 1 – A Bad Fit

A few years ago, we were very excited by the possibility of working with a highly respected local urologist. This physician, who had an extensive practice, was equally excited to work with us. PBRC spoke with him and evaluated his patient base. We found he had a large number of patients with prostate cancer, bladder cancers, etc. Our marketing department was able to locate a good protocol for early bladder cancers. We sent him the protocol and asked him to review it. After he had done so, he told us that he had hundreds of patients who would conform to the inclusion/exclusion criteria and that he probably saw two to three patients per day who might qualify.

We contacted the CRO for the study and PBRC was quickly initiated as a replacement site. In the beginning, the urologist was extremely easy to reach. Our first several patients were screened quickly. He then performed the required cystoscopies and biopsies. Unfortunately, he also treated the early bladder cancers at the same visit. The protocol called for the principal investigator to send the slides to the sponsor to be evaluated prior to treatment. This protocol requirement, however, interrupted his normal routine.

The study coordinator and I sat down with the physician to explain the problems he was creating with his method of treating patients whom he was allegedly also trying to enroll in the protocol. Unfortunately, we were unable to communicate the concept of protocol adherence to him. He continued to follow his usual courses of treatment and therefore, none of the hundreds of patients that he had ever qualified for the study. The physician never could understand why they could not be enrolled. Even though he was a top-notch urologist, he was a poor investigator.

Not surprisingly, we lost the study. The urologist never developed a career in the clinical trials business, and we all learned a valuable and costly lesson. Hence, we developed a system of evaluating physicians before we contract with them to be principal investigators.

Example 2 – A Good Fit

After we had implemented our system of evaluating potential investigators, we documented its success by using it to find two excellent investigators. We identified two local internists who ran a huge practice and had many other internists working for them. We followed our present protocol of testing their level of interest in participating in clinical trials. They quickly returned paperwork and telephone calls and met with us frequently to learn about conducting clinical trials. Over time, we continued to work with them until they wanted to assume the role of investigator.

One partner controlled the business aspect of the practice, while the other oversaw the clinical part of the large internal medicine practice. He had the desire to become a principal investigator, while the more business-oriented partner preferred to remain a sub-investigator. After a few studies, we realized how successful they could be and so did they. Both were extremely motivated.

We eventually created a site around their eight-person practice. They expanded and moved into new office space and dedicated space for our coordinators, research assistants and potential patients. They had the foresight to create a separate waiting room just for research patients.

These two physicians are more the exception than the rule. They are extremely enthusiastic, follow direction well and are able to enroll appropriate patients for the studies. Best of all, they enjoy conducting clinical research and feel a real sense of accomplishment. They also enjoy the prestige that successful clinical trials lend to their practice.

Palm Beach Research Center (PBRC) has developed a booklet and home study materials for potential investigators that detail various FDA guidelines and good clinical practices. Both the director of clinical operations and the research director in-service the potential investigators on these requirements. They also review the protocol with the doctors step-by-step, with special emphasis on the inclusion/exclusion criteria. They explain the Statement of Investigator FDA Form 1572, a legal contract between the investigator and the FDA that outlines the investigator's responsibilities to the FDA, the sponsor, the IRB and to the study subjects. Once potential investigators complete this training and have signed confidentiality agreements in place with PBRC, we allow them to call us with prospective patients who fit various protocols that we forward to the investigators. In addition, we seek their input to help us determine if the protocol under consideration is feasible.

The incentive for physicians is that they have access to medications and treatments that would not otherwise be available to their patients. This access adds value to their practice and helps them attract more patients to it. A good example is a physician who treats arthritis patients. Many of the new arthritis medications that are not available on the market are available through clinical trials. There is a small population of patients whose arthritis is unable to be treated successfully by anything on the market. This physician's ability to offer patients something that is not available on the market not only helps the patient, but it also enhances this physician's reputation in the community. Physicians are also apprised of cutting-edge developments in their field. Lastly, this access helps physicians evaluate how successful these new treatments are through feedback from us and follow-up with the patient.

After a period ranging from a few months to two years of this activity, and after gauging their level of interest, we promote them to the next step, which is becoming a sub-investigator. Eventually, some sub-investigators move on to become principal investigators, and they work within our center under supervision. After we are confident of an investigator's ability to follow good clinical practices, exercise good judgment and be a solid physician, we have discussions with that physician to determine the level of interest in conducting studies at his or her own office.

One source of excellent investigators is retired physicians. Using our system of evaluating potential investigators, we have promoted several into the role of principal investigator. If they have been community leaders, they can bring patients and great prestige to your center. They may not need additional income, but are interested in staying busy and keeping their skills sharp. I have always been impressed with the caliber of these physicians.

Successful Contracting with Investigators

Once we accept a physician as an investigator, we forward an agreement to him or her. The typical sorts of relationship arrangements are listed in Table 2. A sample of some of the agreements described in this chapter can be found in Appendix b.

The "Investigator Agreement" is simple and straightforward and outlines the basic elements of the relationship. It treats the physician as an independent contractor, not as an employee of the site, and it can be used for investigators and sub-investigators. This contract covers both parties for an indefinite period of time, thereby eliminating the need to re-draft the contract for each individual study. The payment schedule for each study is a separate attachment to the contract. Either party can terminate the agreement by giving the other party ninety days' written notice. It also contains a confidentiality clause as well as a statement that the investigator is required to disclose any outside activities or interests that conflict or may conflict with the best interests of the site. An example would be a competing study that the investigator is conducting through a competing site.

Some Types of Contracts Between Sites and Investigators
Investigator Agreement
Consultant Agreement
Confidentiality Agreement

Table 2

An important part of the agreement is a rather benign non-compete section, which lasts for a period of only ninety days following termination of the agreement. This section offers the site a modicum of protection against an investigator who attempts to compete directly or indirectly against the site during that ninety-day period. During this time, it precludes the investigator from contacting the sponsor directly to discuss opportunities about procuring his or her own studies.

Another type of arrangement between a site and an investigator is the "Consultant Agreement." This is an agreement that can be used with an investigator who does not wish to participate in clinical trials as an investigator or sub-investigator, but who is interested in servicing our staff, acting as a resource in his or her area of expertise, and making his or her patients aware of specific protocols. The agreement is straightforward, and is easy to terminate with thirty days' written notice.

The "Confidentiality Agreement" is used with investigators and with other private contractors who, in our judgment, may have the capacity to offer direct competition. It is not uncommon for some sub-investigators to have a hidden agenda of being trained by us, want access to our pharmaceutical contracts and our trained study coordinators, and then aim to lure them away. Although there is no way to stop free enterprise, we attempt to limit this from happening via this agreement.

It includes a restrictive covenant against the contractor contacting the pharmaceutical client(s) or engaging any of the site's employees as employees, consultants or independent contractors for a period of one year following the termination of the contractor's relationship with the site. Some of the sample language appears in Table 3.

Sample Language in the Non-Compete and Confidentiality Agreement

"For a period of one (1) year following the termination of the Contractor's relationship with the site, whether voluntary or involuntary, the Contractor shall not, directly or indirectly, on behalf of the Contractor or any other party, either (a) solicit or offer to provide to any Pharmaceutical Client services of the types provided by the site; or (b) furnish or provide such service to any Pharmaceutical Client. These restrictions shall apply to the Contractor's business and professional activities conducted in the following counties…."

"For a period of one (1) year following the termination of the Contractor's relationship with the site, whether voluntary or involuntary, the Contractor shall not directly or indirectly, on behalf of the Contractor or any other party, engage any of the site's key employees, as employees, consultants, independent contractors or otherwise. As used herein, 'key employee' shall include any person who has been employed by the site at any time within 90 days prior to the termination of the Contractor's relationship with the site, as a coordinator or a regulatory department employee."

Table 3

Coordinators: Make It a Win/Win

The hallmark of a solid, advanced site is one that maintains its study coordinators. The larger, more successful sites seem to have a common philosophy for hiring coordinators. They generally do not advertise these openings. They recruit from within or through networking with individuals known to the industry or known by reliable people working at the site.

The study coordinator is the most valuable player at the site, and once the site finds this MVP, the employment contract should lay out the agreed upon terms in a straightforward, non-threatening way. (See the "Hiring and Retaining Your Study Coordinators" chapter for more on this important position.)

The "Employment Contract" should include the following:

- Term
- Compensation
- Vacation
- Benefits
- Terms under which the contract terminates
- Confidential non-disclosure
- Non-compete clause

Contracting with Other Sites

Along with signing up potential investigators and good study coordinators, the growing site will eventually need to contract with other individual sites, and may also consider creating or participating in a network of sites across the country. Arrangements can take the form of your site contracting with others, or other sites contracting with yours. Whether arrangements are formal or informal, these affiliations can serve to grow your site more quickly by offering access to many studies, and expanding your network of contacts (Table 4).

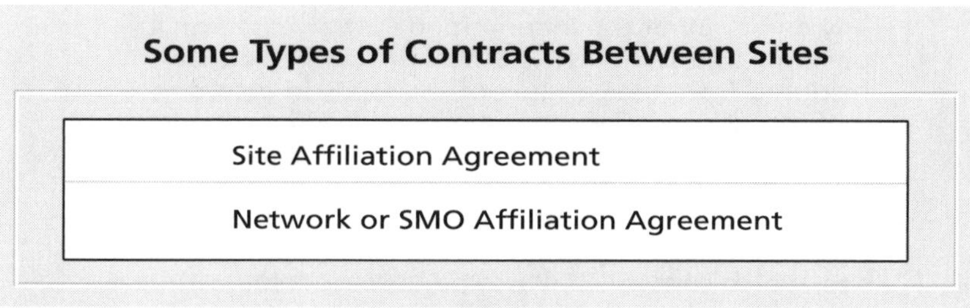

Some Types of Contracts Between Sites
Site Affiliation Agreement
Network or SMO Affiliation Agreement

Table 4

One way for other individual sites to contract with yours is through a "Site Affiliation Agreement." This contract provides that the site interested in contracting with yours ("main site") agrees to a number of stipulations including:

- The affiliated site selects the Principal Investigator who must conduct the research in accordance with applicable policies of the sponsor and the main site.
- The research is to be conducted in accordance with the protocol, and if the affiliated site deviates from it, the affiliated site is to promptly notify the main site and the sponsor in writing of the deviations.
- The site prepares and maintains complete, accurately written records, accounts, notes, reports and data for the research.
- The site prepares and submits to the sponsor all of the original case report forms and electronic files for each patient.
- The site maintains worker's compensation insurance, as well as general liability insurance with combined limits of not less than an amount per occurrence that is required by law in its locale.
- The site maintains an amount of insurance that is usual and customary in its locale per accident for bodily injury, including death and property damage.
- The site certifies that no person involved in the research has been

Sample Language that Indemnifies the Site

Sponsor shall indemnify, defend and hold harmless the site, the institutional review board, the principal investigator, all other persons listed on form 1572, including without limitation, approved clinical investigators and personnel working under their direct supervision and any other affiliates involved in the study, and their officers, directors, shareholders, owners, employees, agent and subcontractors (hereinafter referred to as the "Indemnified Parties") against any rightful or wrongful causes of action, claims, demands, actions, suits, costs, liabilities, expenses, damages, and fees, including attorney's fees (a Claim) brought against any one or all of the Indemnified Parties based on a personal injury, disease, sickness or death allegedly resulting from the conduct of the study in accordance with the protocol or the use of any product submitted by the sponsor. The site shall promptly notify sponsor upon receipt of notice of any Claim. Sponsor shall assume the defense and costs of such Claim, utilizing attorneys chosen by sponsor with the consent of the site, which consent shall not be unreasonably withheld. The site and sponsor shall fully cooperate and aid in all defenses under this section ... This section shall survive any termination of this agreement."

Table 5

debarred under section 306a (mandatory debarment) or 306b (permissive debarment) of the Federal Food, Drug and Cosmetic Act.*

The agreement also includes standard clauses such as those pertaining to compensation, confidentiality, and rights of both parties to terminate the agreement.

By entering into a "Network or SMO Affiliation Agreement," the growing site gains several advantages. Generally, by associating with a network, the site gains access to marketing, management and budgeting services. Either the site or the network can provide regulatory functions. The site can provide its own coordinators. Budgetary issues are generally part of the agreement, sometimes as an attached exhibit.

Site Indemnification

Over the past few years, sites have actively pursued site indemnification, which refers to the sponsor or CRO holding them harmless against any causes of action, claims or suits brought against them resulting from the conduct of a study in accordance with the protocol. At the same time, sponsors and CROs have stepped up the pressure on investigative sites to indemnify them against product liability claims. In so doing, the sponsors and CROs attempt to shift their risk exposure to the sites. The larger, more sophisticated sites are savvy to this and will turn down studies if the indemnification section of the contract cannot be satisfactorily negotiated. Table 5 shows some acceptable sample indemnification language.

It is our experience at PBRC that more recently, sponsors and CROs are trying to reduce the degree of indemnification they extend to the site. For this reason, we suggest carrying extra umbrella insurance in the form of a malpractice policy. At PBRC, we have an umbrella policy that covers the entire site. This type of insurance is available from niche players that specialize in insurance products for clinical research organizations. Umbrella policies may also be available from these same insurance carriers.

All parties involved with the conduct of a study at your site need indemnification. This includes physicians, students, volunteers, vendors and hospitals. In fact, some sponsors require the sites to provide proof of this coverage. We require all of our principal and sub-investigators to carry their own malpractice policies. One exception to this is that we sometimes carry malpractice policies on the few physicians working within our site who do not carry their own, namely the retired physicians.

* The FDA Debarment List refers to firms or individuals convicted of a felony under federal law for conduct (by a firm) relating to the development or approval of any abbreviated drug application; or (an individual convicted) for conduct relating to development or approval of any drug product, or otherwise relating to any drug product under the Federal Food, Drug, and Cosmetic Act. *http://www.fda.gov/ora/compliance_ref/debar/default.htm*

We also require the nurses of our investigators to carry malpractice policies. Nurse malpractice policies are generally inexpensive, costing a few hundred dollars per year. The principal, sub-investigator and nurse malpractice policies need to be reviewed carefully because some of them specifically exclude coverage for research activities, or fail to mention coverage for clinical research. If so, the policy needs to be modified to include this type of coverage.

Additional items to consider for indemnification purposes appear in Table 6. Also, the indemnification should survive the termination of the project and termination of the contract because of the possibility of patients coming back years later with a problem that they believe is related to the clinical trial in which they participated. A typical indemnification period lasts for two years following study completion. The key is to have the site and personnel indemnified for a period of time roughly equal to the statute of limitations for the surfacing of an adverse event.

When drafting the indemnification section of the agreement, you will want to consider the sponsor's financial position. It is important to make sure that the company is able to back up the negotiated indemnification. Financial information on large pharmaceutical companies is easily obtained

Additional Items to Consider for Indemnification Purposes
Indemnification against claims from patients who were given the placebo or the comparator, or used rescue medications, IV fluids or any other substances relating to the study
Indemnification against adverse events arising from washout periods
Indemnification against adverse events arising from diagnostic, surgical or emergency procedures
There is a reasonable reporting period for the indemnification "event" such as 30 days, as opposed to one or two days.
Check the statute of limitations in your state to make sure that the indemnification will last for a substantial period following the end of the study, at least two years, for example.

Table 6

because they are generally publicly traded and/or appear in Dunn & Bradstreet. It may be more difficult to determine the financial position of smaller sponsors. You may wish to contact your attorney to help determine that these sponsors are not shell companies with limited liability and assets and that they are able to support the indemnification you are seeking.

Indemnification is extending to hospitals. A number of them require a letter of indemnification from the sponsor. Securing this letter from the sponsor can be challenging, but it is a worthwhile effort if your site has an opportunity to participate in a good inpatient study.

A number of sponsors are increasingly asking investigators to hold them harmless from claims arising from investigator error. This is known as "cross indemnification." An example would be an investigator missing an inner cerebral bleed and mistaking it for a migraine headache. This is a drastic example of an activity that falls under the purview of the investigator's responsibility, not the sponsor's. A less extreme example is when the investigator is unsuccessfully treating a patient with the study drug for acute sinusitis because in fact, the patient has chronic allergic rhinitis. Some language addressing cross indemnification appears in Table 7.

The underwriters that provide insurance policies for the investigators usually name the pharmaceutical sponsor as an additional insured to the investigator's policy. Therefore, the insurance company of the primary

Sample Language Indemnifying Sponsor from Investigator Error

This indemnity shall not apply to any claim which is attributable to:
(a) the failure of the principal investigator or any other personnel engaged by the principal investigator to assist in the conduct of the study to (i) adhere to all material terms of the protocol or any written instructions relative to the use of any product(s) used in the performance of the study (deviations arising out of necessity and not contributing to the injury or affecting study validity shall not be considered a failure to adhere to the protocol) or (ii) comply with all material applicable FDA or other governmental requirements or
(b) any grossly negligent, willfully malfeasant or intentionally wrongful act or omission of the site, the principal investigator or any other personnel of the site directly involved in the study.

Table 7

investigator provides protection to the pharmaceutical company in the event of a lawsuit or any other action against the investigator for negligence or malpractice. In this way, the primary investigator can cross-indemnify the sponsor. Conversely, the site should request that the pharmaceutical sponsor name the investigator's site as an additional insured to its policy. This is true cross-indemnification. It is important that the site, a corporate entity, be named in the sponsor's policy as opposed to naming the investigator in order to avoid putting the investigator's personal assets at risk.

Example 3 – The Importance of Being Indemnified

Sometimes people have complications or side effects from the study medication or even the current medications that are used as the control for the study. For example, a study that one of the other sites did was using nonsteroidal anti-inflammatory medications to treat osteoarthritis. One of their patients developed a significant ulcer and a gastrointestinal bleed from this ulcer. The patient was subsequently hospitalized and needed blood transfusions and emergency surgery. This is not an uncommon complication for this class of drug, which the patient had been on previously for osteoarthritis. Unfortunately, the patient did not see it that way and went straight to a lawyer after getting out of the hospital. Luckily, the site had indemnification through the sponsor and was able to use the sponsor's insurance company, which provided legal counsel to take care of this problem. It was resolved without going to court and taken care of without the site's incurring any expense because of the indemnification agreement.

The site also carried its own indemnity insurance in case the situation progressed to a point beyond what the company would have covered. Because the initial complaint was that the patient was not being treated properly, the patient's attorney felt that the physician at the site should have recognized the signs of a gastrointestinal bleed prior to the patient's hospitalization. The attorney was trying to split representation and not only sued the sponsor but also sued the investigator separately. Fortunately, the investigator had his own indemnity insurance in addition to being indemnified from the company and was therefore protected.

In Review

The best way for investigative sites to grow is by reaching out to their community for clinical partners, namely investigators, study coordinators and other established sites. Expanding the site's network of contacts raises the site's visibility and may increase its chances of being considered for a broader range of appropriate studies. Before deciding to contract with a new investigator, it is wise to evaluate the willingness of that physician to follow protocols and learn about good clinical practice.

Establishing relationships with clinical partners consistently means putting contracts or letters of agreement in place that describe the expectations for each party. Developing templated agreements and contracts can save the site much time and money, as these kinds of agreements into which it will enter tend to be the same.

When sites contract with sponsors, a key issue today is indemnification. Sites are seeking to be indemnified from claims arising from problems resulting from studies, and sponsors want to be indemnified from problems relating to their products. Hospitals want to be indemnified by sponsors if the study has an inpatient component. Negotiating indemnification can be sensitive and difficult, with both sides wanting to be indemnified from the mistakes of the other. Although sites may be well advised to walk away from contracts in which they are not properly indemnified, it is reasonable for sites to assume responsibility for errors made by the investigator. These errors may take several forms, including but not limited to, misdiagnosis, protocol violation leading to adverse events or malfeasance.

The site needs to maintain insurance that includes coverage for clinical research activities. All parties involved in the study should be insured. A number of insurance carriers specialize in this type of malpractice coverage.

References

[i] "Where we are and where we're going," *The Monitor*, Association of Clinical Research Professionals, James W. Maloy et al., Summer 2000, p. 25.

[ii] "Investigator Scrutiny and Certification," *The Monitor*, The Association of Clinical Research Professionals, James W. Maloy et al, Summer 2001, p. 31.

CHAPTER 7

Budgeting

- Getting Started on the Budgeting Process
- Contracting with Sponsors and CROs
- The Cash Flow Problem
- Tracking Cash Flow
- Profitability of the Site
- In Review

As I've noted, the previous six chapters discuss growing the infrastructure of your investigative site. The decision to expand is informed by several criteria, including recognition that the site is too crowded or too bogged down with work, staff is overly stressed and the site cannot accept more studies without adding infrastructure. The next steps are implementing and maintaining proper operating controls and processes.

In the coming chapters, I'll discuss maintaining proper operating controls: prudent budgeting, investing time and money in improving office systems and electronic medical records and other e-solutions. Key operating processes revolve around patient recruitment, enrollment and protection. The last chapter of the book details how to value your site before selling it. Selling your site may be an important exit strategy down the road. The ramifications of selling to different buyers are also explored.

Once a site is positioned to accept more studies, the success of that site hinges largely on the negotiation of contracts with profitable budgets. Although some dedicated sites report annual increases in gross revenues in the 19% to 20% range,[i] developing profitable budgets is always a challenge. Competition for studies is stiff, as the number of sites is now estimated in excess of 10,000.[ii] Grant size is increasing a mere 3% to 4% annually, while overhead costs rise and the number of procedures per protocol is growing by 8% to 10% each year.[iii] When adjusted for inflation, fees per patient were flat between 1990 and 2000 (Figure 1).[iv]

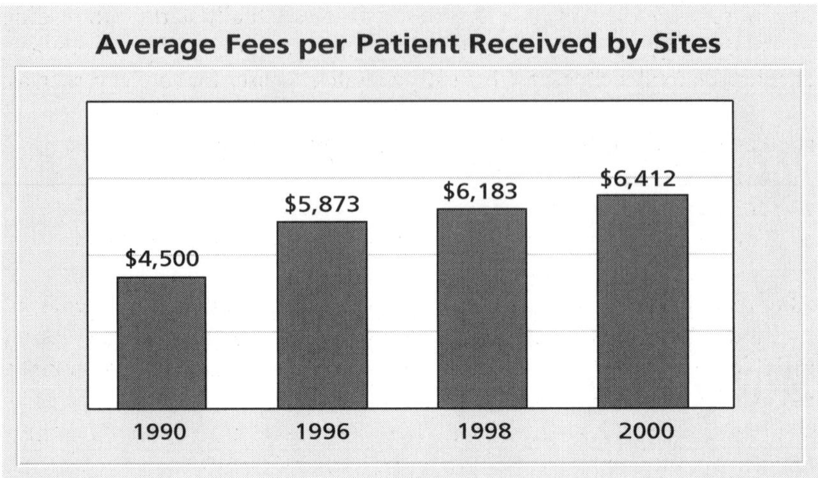

Figure 1 Source: CenterWatch

Gross revenues are on the rise because sites are accepting more business. In 2000, sponsors and Clinical Research Organizations (CROs) hiked spending on clinical grants to investigators by 18%, reaching an estimated total of $4.52 billion.[v] Translating additional revenue into profits takes planning and an ability to determine if a budget proposed by a sponsor or a CRO is reasonable. This is particularly important for growing sites that are adding a costly infrastructure because more study dollars will now be earmarked to support the expanded overhead. It may seem counterintuitive, but the most profitable sites are those doing a handful of studies because they have little overhead to support.

Getting Started on the Budgeting Process

Developing and negotiating successful study budgets is truly an art that is refined through experience. Knowing your costs, knowing what is involved in a specific protocol and anticipating the unexpected are skills acquired through the conduct of many studies in various therapeutic areas.

Clinical trials budgets generally fall into three categories:

- A fixed budget offered by the sponsor or CRO to the site

- A budget proposed by the site to a sponsor or CRO seeking competitive bids
- A budget developed by the site for a protocol whose budget needs are unclear because the sponsor has never held a trial of its type before

Regardless of budget type, the budgeting process actually starts with reading the study protocol. This offers a sense of the complexity of the study and enables you to identify items that will generate expenses for your site, such as:

- The number of study visits required and the estimated length of each visit
- The number and types of procedures involved
- The estimated length of time needed to obtain informed consent

After reading the protocol, the next step is to evaluate the appropriateness of the study for your site. Answering a series of questions, such as those found in Table 1, can help organize your thinking about the study. You will want to pay particular attention to studies with challenging study inclusion/exclusion criteria such as those targeting diabetics controlled using insulin pumps filled by family members; wound studies seeking healthy patients with no other problems but bed sores; herpes zoster studies in search of subjects who have had an outbreak of shingles within a 24-hour period and have not taken any pain medication; or AIDS studies wanting treatment-naïve patients.

If preliminary reaction to a protocol is generally positive, additional evaluations should be done to estimate the time commitment and the associated costs of procedures for each study visit. A flow chart of study visits can be used for this purpose (Table 2).

Once the activities of each visit are charted, the next step is to assign the costs for those activities. In your geographic area, you will need to know the costs for:

- A medical history
- A physical examination
- A chest x-ray
- An electrocardiogram
- A complete blood count (CBC)
- A blood draw, followed by processing, packing and shipping the blood

The next step is to evaluate the cost of time spent by the study coordinator, research assistants, laboratory staff and office personnel. At PBRC, we estimate this by reviewing historical averages of time spent completing specific tasks. For example, we know that it typically takes one hour for the investigator to review inclusion/exclusion criteria with the patient, 60 to 90 minutes for the coordinator to review the informed consent form with the

Sample Evaluation Form for Study Feasibility

1. The CRO or Sponsor ____________
2. Protocol Number ____________
3. Principal Investigator ____________
4. Number of subjects needed for study ____________
5. Is study schedule within appropriate time lines? ☐ Yes ☐ No
6. Do we have facilities and staff for this? ☐ Yes ☐ No
7. If no, can we obtain staff and facility for this? ☐ Yes ☐ No
8. Do we have any competing studies? ☐ Yes ☐ No
9. Any special requirements for study? ☐ Yes ☐ No
10. If yes, what equipment is required? ____________
11. Procedures? ☐ Yes ☐ No
12. Which procedures? ____________
13. Do we need added sub-investigators? ☐ Yes ☐ No

    Who? ____________
14. Should we consider this study? ☐ Yes ☐ No

Investigator's comments ____________

Coordinator (Name) ____________

Coordinator's comments ____________

Director of Clinical Operations (Name) ____________

Director's comments ____________

Table 1

Sample Study Flow chart

Visit Type	Screen	Baseline		Treatment				Final			Surgical Follow-up	Safety Follow-up
Visit Number	1	2a**	2b***	3	4	5	6	7+	8a	8b+	9a	9b
Visit Time (weeks)	-2 to -5	-2 to -5	-1 to -4	0	1	4	8	11	12	13	14	16
Procedure												
Medical History	X											
Physical Exam	X					X	X		X			
Vital Signs*	X			X	X	X	X		X			
Height	X			X		X			X			
Weight	X								X			
12 Lead ECG	X											

* Vital Signs: Blood pressure (standing, sitting and supine), heart rate, respiratory rate, temperature

** Hematology: Hemoglobin, hematocrit, RBC with indices, WBC with differential and platelet count

*** Fasting Blood Chemistry: sodium, potassium, chloride, bicarbonate or carbon dioxide, glucose, BUN, creatinine, calcium, phosphorous, uric acid, total protein, albumin, A/B ratio, cholesterol, total bilirubin, triglycerides, AST (GOT), ALT (GPT), lactic dehydrogenase (LDH), alkaline phosphatase, CPK

Table 2

patient and thirty minutes to draw blood, collect urine samples and complete associated paperwork. Although physical examinations are generally completed in 40 to 60 minutes, more time is factored in for arthritis studies that require joint assessments or stroke studies that use global assessment tools. Table 3 shows examples of time needed to complete specific tasks.

After the cost of procedures and labor is computed from the flow chart (Table 2), add a 25% overhead to cover fixed costs such as rent, utilities, insurance, office supplies, employee benefits, the cost of dry ice for shipment and off-site record storage. Softer overhead costs include the time needed to meet with pre-study site selectors, develop a screening form, screen patients, complete case report forms, complete serious adverse event (SAE) reports, prepare document packages for IRB submission and submit data to the sponsor or CRO. These overhead costs highlight the reality that even the best accounting tools may do little to pin down real costs beyond those that are fixed. There are no accounting tricks to reflect the amount of time study coordinators or other staff spend on the telephone attempting to track down patients to avoid missing certain windows or traveling between physician offices to coordinate a study at multiple local sites. There is no way to estimate exactly how much time will be spent making photocopies, faxing materials and speaking with monitors or sponsors' representatives to discuss particulars of the protocol or reviewing patient diaries. These are predictable activities but the time spent doing them varies from study to study. One way to make an educated guess is to review time sheets from previous studies of a similar nature. They can serve to highlight the amount of time spent on revenue-producing and non-revenue-producing (administrative) tasks.

Estimated Times Needed to Complete Specific Tasks
30 minutes for blood draw
60–90 minutes to review informed consent form with the patient
30 minutes for EKG
40–60 minutes or more for history and physical
30–90 minutes for follow-up visit
2–3 hours to follow patient for endoscopy procedures

Table 3

There are some additional points to consider in the development of a budget. These appear in Table 4.

This detailed budgeting exercise is necessary to help you determine the anticipated costs for each study and the number of enrolled patients needed to reach the break-even point. Assuming that your costs are properly calculated, you will be able to estimate the profitability of the study based on the level of enrollment success. To maintain that profitability, obtain written approval for payment from the sponsor or CRO before incurring additional study costs not included in the initial budget.

A careful approach is advised whether the sponsor or CRO provides a fixed budget, or whether you develop a budget to submit as part of a study proposal. Once the budget is developed, it can always be modified. To avoid overbidding, and precluding your site from consideration, you will want to ask the sponsor or CRO for a hint about the budget range it is expecting. This knowledge helps you to determine if the study makes financial sense for your site.

Additional Points to Consider When Developing a Study Budget
Obtain coordinator input
Propose that the sponsor or CRO be financially responsible for the cost of the laboratory tests when a central laboratory is not used. (When a central laboratory is used, it is generally understood that the sponsor is financially responsible for the cost of the lab work.)
Propose that the sponsor or CRO be financially responsible for the cost of obtaining patients' medical records as most offices charge a fee for providing them.
Propose that remuneration not be affected by natural disasters or occurrence of serious adverse events.
A proposed budget should be valid for only ninety (90) days.

Table 4

Budgets presented by CROs or sponsors that are allegedly "fixed" can sometimes be negotiated if they seem to be inadequate. The best way to do this is to calculate your costs as accurately as possible and demonstrate your track record of success in the therapeutic area of interest. Sites with less experience and a shorter track record may not be able to negotiate from the same position of strength as older, more established sites. This is particularly true if a site is young, if it is entering a new therapeutic area or if it is working with a new sponsor or CRO. If the proposed fixed budget from the sponsor is truly inadequate, it is best to walk away from the study.

Oftentimes sponsors will approach inexperienced investigators who will accept the budget. The budget will seem generous to them, even though it is not. Early on, you realize that you are accepting a budget for a study that will end up losing money and force you to subsidize the sponsor's research. Most investigators do not know what their true costs are. By breaking down all aspects of the study you can figure out your costs.

Certain studies, such as in-hospital studies or studies that require patients in certain populations, such as dialysis patients or patients with chronic pulmonary disease, may end up with a lot of serious adverse events or adverse events. This will take up a great deal of your coordinator's time, as well as that of the rest of your staff and could easily soak up the profit.

The other problem with some fixed budgets is that they don't allow for screen failures. Some studies have very strict criteria and may have a lot of screen failures. If you spend your time bringing in patients, interviewing them, having them sign consents, then sending out initial blood work, only to then have the patient fail because of some value on the blood work, you will again soak up all the profit.

These are items to include when expanding a "fixed" budget:

- Payment to move records in and out of storage
- Payment for advertising associated with patient recruitment initiatives

The budget for patient recruitment should be separately negotiated. Developing a plan designed to reach patient enrollment targets is critical to the success of a study and to the success of your site. By the mid-1990s, sponsors started to understand the importance of sites making detailed patient recruitment plans and are now often willing to commit dollars toward that effort.[vi] Making a patient recruitment budget requires an understanding of the therapeutic area in question and a recognition that different approaches are needed for different therapeutic areas. Recruiting for an osteoporosis study may require different tactics than recruiting patients for an asthma trial.

As the site continues to grow, there should be more of a delineation between the business and the clinical side of the business. Because physicians generally are not trained in budgetary matters, it is better to leave these tasks to people who are. At the advanced site, physicians should be focusing almost exclusively on taking care of patients, not budgets.

Contracting with Sponsors and CROs

It is useful to have a basic contract, or Master Agreement, in place between your site and each CRO and sponsor with which you expect to do business. Some sponsors have developed boilerplate forms, but your site may want to develop its own for use as needed. Once a basic contract is in place, separate agreements for individual studies can become attachments to the basic contract. The separate agreement addresses specifics of a study such as issues surrounding patient recruitment, or the need for special procedures or equipment.

A Master Agreement sets forth rights and obligations of both parties and includes a number of standard contract elements such as:

- Scope of work
- Reporting of data and adverse events
- Monitoring of the studies by the sponsor or CRO
- Budget (Table 5)
- Termination of agreement
- Indemnification of the site (see Chapter 6)

This boilerplate agreement will direct your relationship and will enable you to avoid re-negotiating the same terms repeatedly as new study opportunities arise. This saves time and money and may limit the ongoing involvement of the sponsor's or CRO's legal department.

Suggested Budget Language in a Master Agreement Between a Site and CRO or Sponsor

"The total payments which sponsor shall make to the site to complete the study, including the number of patients specified in the protocol, are as provided in Exhibit A attached hereto and made a part hereof. If fewer or more than the anticipated number of patients complete the study, payments will be prorated as provided in Exhibit A or in such other equitable manner as shall be mutually agreed. Final payment to be made at the earlier of (a) the time at which (i) the last study patient visit has been completed, (ii) all unused experimental drug has been accounted for utilizing sponsor's accounting procedures, (iii) all inquiries reasonably and timely made by sponsor with respect to the study have been satisfactorily answered and (iv) all case report forms have been completed and supplied to sponsor; or (b) 60 days after notification to sponsor of the completion of all case report forms."

Table 5

The Cash Flow Problem

Once the budget is negotiated, and a clinical study begins, the next challenge for the growing site is handling the inevitable cash flow problem. There are various reasons why maintaining positive cash flow can be a significant challenge. See Table 6 for the key reasons.

When a site is expanding, one of the places where a site underestimates costs is in the area of study startup. We have found that expenses for study startup average in the $5,000 to $6,000 range. These include:

- Time spent procuring the study, such as development of a proposal, and time spent with pre-study site selector
- Preparation of paperwork necessary for the study, including tracking forms and screening forms
- Regulatory submissions
- Time spent for study initiation—typically an entire day
- Time spent training hospital staff, nursing and pharmacy personnel, if study has an inpatient component

Reasons for a Cash Flow Problem
Startup costs were underestimated.
Site failed to negotiate any upfront payment for startup costs.
The sponsor or CRO is slow to pay.
Site failed to negotiate payment for work done on screen failures.
The sponsor cancels the study.
The site decides to withdraw from the study.

Table 6

Recently, some sponsors and CROs have become more inclined to provide upfront money earmarked for startup costs. Typically, these sums are in the $1500 to $2000 range and may be seen as an attempt to defray the cost of initial regulatory submissions made by a site to a local institutional review board (IRB). These upfront dollars must be requested, as sponsors and CROs do not forward them automatically. If the sponsor opts for a central IRB, the sponsor will pay those fees directly; however, upfront money can still be requested to offset other startup costs.

The fact that some sponsors and CROs are often slow to pay is a key contributor to cash flow problems. While some sponsors pay in a timely fashion, it is not unusual for larger sponsors and CROs to take 180 to 250 days to make payments, even though contracts may call for sponsors or CROs to make quarterly payments or milestone payments triggered by events such as the randomization of the first five patients, for example. The delay may be attributed to the fact that some sponsors or CROs may decline to make a payment until the monitor comes to retrieve the data. This could take months. Another reason for payment delay is that some sponsors or CROs have slow internal systems for signing payment vouchers.

It is also commonplace for some sponsors or CROs to hold back 10% to 20% of the negotiated budget amount until the study database is locked and all queries are completed. When negotiating the budget, you should request that this final payment be contingent upon completion of all queries at your site, and not for all sites participating in the study.

I also suggest negotiating specific milestones in the study contract that trigger each payment. Besides any startup funds you can procure, you will also want to request a second payment after study initiation and the enrollment of the first five patients. Together, the startup and second payments could total 20% of the study budget. If the total enrollment target is twenty patients, another 20% could be billed following the enrollment of ten patients, a third 20% after fifteen patients are enrolled, a fourth 20% after enrollment is completed and a final 20% payment when the last case report form (CRF) is completed. You will want to request additional payment in the event your site over-enrolls the study. Because over-enrollment means that your site has exceeded its patient recruitment goals, you may be able to negotiate a higher budget per patient if the study warrants it.

Some sites add penalties to overdue payments; however, most fear that attempting to penalize a sponsor or CRO could result in alienating or losing that client. An alternative might be to empower someone at your site with responsibility for calling companies every day to remind those employees with authority to release checks to forward overdue funds. In addition, sending monthly invoices to sponsors and CROs is a good idea because the negotiated payments are generally past due for the startup costs and for the reaching of milestones that have been confirmed by study monitors. Sometimes, the contract prohibits the mailing of invoices. In those cases, it is best to place a telephone call.

Another cause of cash flow problems stems from failure by sites to request payment for screen failures. Some studies have screening and washout periods lasting several weeks. If a patient fails the screening process, this may happen following a number of patient visits, involving much staff and investigator time. It is reasonable to request in writing to be compensated for this effort.

Example 1 – Study with a High Rate of Screen Failures

Several years ago, we conducted a phase III hypertension study directly with a sponsor. Unbeknownst to us, this sponsor was notorious for not paying the full contract and for taking an unusually long time to make payments.

This hypertension study was extremely difficult to fill. Not only were patients hard to find due to tough inclusion/exclusion criteria, there was also a six-week screening and washout period. We screened 15 to 20 patients for each person enrolled. We were fortunate to enroll six patients, but they came at a tremendous cost. We had patients who completed the screening phase as well as those who were in the study for a few weeks before becoming screen failures. We were told verbally, both by the monitor and by the sponsor, that we would be paid for these screen failures.

When it was time for payment, the sponsor had a new medical director. Because he had not been privy to our previous verbal agreement, we had to plead our case to him for seven months before receiving partial payment. This is an example of a study in which the budget appeared generous and profitable but wasn't, due to this screen failure issue. Consider screen failures in the budgeting process and be certain to put this in writing.

Cancellation of studies by sponsors is another source of cash flow problems. A study may be canceled for any number of reasons, such as the release of new toxicology information, safety problems, intolerable side effects or lack of efficacy. It is important to plan for this eventuality because if the site has already started the study, it may have spent 20% to 30% of the study budget for startup costs. Compensation for this effort is required to maintain profitability; therefore, a cancellation fee should be considered based upon the length of time involved and the dollars invested in the study as determined by the number of procedures completed, number of patients randomized and number of patients completed. Furthermore, the canceled study leaves a hole in the schedule with little opportunity to generate other immediate business.

There are rare instances when a site may choose to terminate a study. Sometimes the site discovers that the study is not a good one due to problems arising from the medication or from patients. The site should retain the right to terminate a project with just compensation if significant adverse events or other types of serious problems arise. Determining just compensation emerges from the number and cost of study procedures conducted up to the point of termination, plus the overhead allocated based on the percentage of patient enrollment reached and the study of completed subjects.

Example 2 – Canceling a Study Because Patients Suffered Too Many Adverse Events

A large southern site participated in a phase II study for a new type of pain medication that many believed was going to revolutionize the world of pain treatment. The study nurse and investigator were extremely enthusiastic about participating in this study, as were the directors of several major pain centers in the immediate area.

The site started the study with great anticipation but after several months of having patients pass out or suffer extreme complications, such as falling into tables or going into semi-comatose states with normal dosing, the investigator and coordinators questioned the use of the medication. The patients, who had been treated for years with narcotics, were chronic pain patients with multiple ailments. A significant percentage of the patients used breakthrough medication and returned to their narcotics. Patients were calling the site on an almost daily basis, and after many adverse events, the lead study coordinator was experiencing extreme stress. Needless to say, the site wanted to drop the study in spite of its generous budget. The investigator and coordinators concluded that this was not a worthwhile medication, as did the monitors from a private monitoring company who had expressed the same concerns. The site later learned that many other sites were facing the same challenges.

The site notified the sponsor of its intent to withdraw from the study and was eventually paid for visits completed up to that point, including the termination visit.

Tracking Cash Flow

Because maintaining positive cash flow is so critical to the survival of a site, it should be tracked carefully each month. We use a special tool for this purpose. We track monthly expenses and monthly incoming revenues earned and to be received (Table 7). In addition, we keep a master study list that identifies all upcoming, ongoing and completed studies. For each study, the list shows the number of patients enrolled, number of patients completed and the time frames for study startup, enrollment, randomization and patient completion. The list enables us to see how close we are to reaching milestones that trigger payments.

In addition to tracking cash flow from completed and current studies, we also make monthly projections about cash flow for upcoming trials. These projections include estimates for studies on which we are currently bidding as well as those on which we plan to bid. It can often take anywhere from three to eight months to receive payment for ongoing studies, so forecasting offers a suggestion of when you will have sufficient cash to fund new studies while paying for existing ones. This exercise also enables you to estimate profit margins. With this information, you can figure out how many studies and which studies to pursue that will lead to your reaching your desired profit margins. Marketing and sales tactics can be planned to support these goals.

Sample Cash Flow Sheet

Contracted Studies	Total # of Pts.	Total # Still in Run-in	Total # Randomized	Rev. Per Compensation Patient	Expected Budget Based on Enrollment	Revenue Earned to Date	Amount Rec'd to Date	Amount Still Owed
Protocol 1	59	N/A	35	$4,615	$161,525	$137,470	$13,470	$124,470
Protocol 2	3	N/A	2	$3,100	$6,200	$1,300	$9,300	($8,000)
Protocol 3	34	N/A	25	$3,700	$92,500	$102,275	$30,130	$72,145
Protocol 4	6	N/A	5	$3,850	$19,250	$5,900	$7,700	($1,800)
Protocol 5	12	N/A	11	$6,652	$73,172	$26,244	$6,452	$19,792
Protocol 6	6	N/A	3	$7,825	$23,475	$8,000	$7,825	$175
Protocol 7	26	N/A	24	$4,300	$103,200	$69,200	$22,650	$46,500
Protocol 8	65	25	16	$3,317	$53,072	$57,208	$7,960	$49,248

Table 7

Profitability of the Site

Investigative sites have high fixed costs, high overhead and unpredictable cash flow, yet well-managed sites are turning a profit. As mentioned earlier in the book, respondents to the 2000 CenterWatch survey of forty-five dedicated sites forecasted 11% to 15% net operating profit margins on average annual revenues of $1.63 million. Nearly 90% of respondents reported that they are profitable. A 1999 CenterWatch survey of 103 investigative sites shows an 11% net operating profit margin of $115,000 on annual gross revenues of $1.06 million. Revenues and expenses broke down as shown in Table 8.[vii]

At Palm Beach Research Center, physician compensation as a percentage of net revenue is less than the 30% to 35% shown in the survey because we use a different paradigm to create long-term win/win situations with our investigators. To achieve this, we consider the Medicare allowable reimbursement rates for certain procedures such as medical histories, physicals, EKGs, pulmonary function tests, etc., and we pay the physicians 100%, 110% or 120% of the allowable rates, depending upon negotiations. This is in lieu of paying them a percentage of the overall budget. This is a win/win situation because generally to perform these procedures, private physicians receive only 70% to 90% of Medicare allowable reimbursements.

In addition, we spend 14% of net revenue on patient recruitment and patient information, which is double the average shown in Table 8. This expenditure has resulted in our ability to reach enrollment targets more quickly, leading to the faster reaching of payment milestones and, sometimes, over-enrolling. For example, we enrolled 80 patients in an abrasion study when the original contract called for 40 patients; we enrolled 60 patients in a migraine headache study in three months, whereas the original contract was for 25 patients; and we enrolled 279 patients in eight months for a medication being tested for osteoarthritis of the hip and knee, whereas the original contract was for 100 patients.

Income Statement for an Investigative Site (Survey Results)

Gross Revenue	$1,060,123
Lab Fees, Subject Compensation	$50,000 (5%)
Net Revenue	$1,010,123
Marketing and Sales	
Patient Recruitment	$70,000 (7%)
General Marketing	$50,000 (5%)
General and Administrative	
Salaries (with M.D. compensation)	$575,000 (57%)*
Meetings, Conferences, Training, Certification	$45,000 (4%)
Rent	$80,000 (8%)
Other	$75,000 (7%)
Operating Profit	**$115,123 (11%)**

* Physician compensation is typically 30% to 35% of net revenues.

Table 8

Source: CenterWatch

We also contract with thought leaders in specialty fields to provide expertise in various therapeutic areas to maintain a market edge. For example, a prominent rheumatologist with teaching and writing credentials is the director of that specialty for our site. He provides in-services for our staff, utilizes his patients for our studies and helps select protocols. Although this is an additional expense that might eat away at profit margins, it is more than offset by the ready access we gain to patients for rheumatology-related studies and the level of knowledge he offers.

Using these techniques has allowed us to reach net operating profit margins in excess of the 11% average shown in the survey. Staying profitable remains an exercise in careful watching of cash flow as profits are being squeezed from tight budgets involving the increase in the number of procedures per study, slow pay from CROs and sponsors and stiffer competition due to the growth in the number of sites.

In Review

The importance of careful budgeting is critical to the growing site and to older, more established sites. Unless you take the time to pin down the fixed costs and estimate the softer costs and time commitments required for successful completion of a study, there is no way to know if a proposed study will be profitable for your site. Forms to track incoming cash flow and outgoing expenditures are crucial tools. They serve as guides to help determine whether you will be able to meet your payroll, and other fixed costs, and whether you can afford to invest in the startup of a new study. Approximately 20% of study expenses are spent during study startup. These forms can also help you anticipate when you will need to dip into your line of credit.

Many newer sites that are not prepared financially are hit hard during startup and screening phases because they are not aware of how long it takes some CROs and sponsors to pay for services rendered. It is hard to fathom that small investigative sites are subsidizing large billion-dollar sponsors in their research efforts, often by working for six months or longer without getting paid. Once a site has a regular flow of studies, the impact of these long waits is somewhat offset by a regular flow of funds from earlier studies. However, in down cycles, or when a site is first expanding, these long periods of irregular cash flow will truly test the most determined investigators. It is important to plan for this eventuality through organizing the budgeting process.

References

[i] "Uphill Growth for Dedicated Sites," *CenterWatch*, Vol. 7, Issue 12, December 2000, p. 5.

[ii] CenterWatch *Fact Book*, 2000.

[iii] Op. cit., *CenterWatch*, December 2000, p. 6.

[iv] Ibid., *CenterWatch*, December 2000, p. 6.

[v] "Grant Market to Exceed $4 Billion in 2000," *CenterWatch*, Vol. 7, Issue 11, November 2000, p. 1.

[vi] *A Guide to Patient Recruitment: Today's Best Practices and Proven Strategies*, Diana L. Anderson, Ph.D., CenterWatch, Inc., 2001, pp. 13-14.

[vii] "Sites Prosper...but Financial Health Threatened," *CenterWatch*, Vol. 7, Issue 1, January 2000, p. 11.

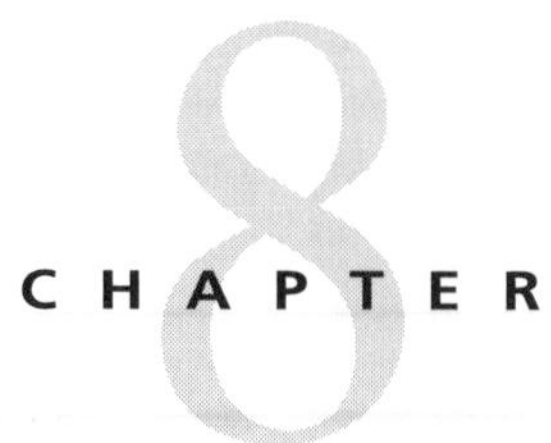

CHAPTER 8

Improving Office Systems

- Telephone Screens, Sign-In Sheets, Universal Source Documents, etc.
- Patient Records and Logs
- Tracking Patient Windows
- Expand the Filing System and Plan for Record Retention and Storage
- Use Management Tools
- Use Office Equipment to Grow the Site
- In Review

This chapter explores the nuts and bolts of office systems needed to streamline the complexity of required clinical trials paperwork. Once these systems are in place, there will be improved study documentation and smoother operations, leaving the staff better positioned to offer good customer service.

Every step of study conduct at the investigative site level seems to require paperwork, beginning with study startup documentation, such as FDA Statement of Investigator Form 1572, the signing of protocol amendments, financial disclosure forms, investigator CVs and all IRB documentation, continuing through to study closeout. The regulatory responsibilities and sponsor requirements for the documenting of all clinical and administrative tasks relating to these study activities can be daunting (Table 1). Breaking down the required paperwork into steps renders the tasks less overwhelming and turns regulatory recordkeeping requirements into more routine activity.

A few of the various processes that need to be implemented are:

- Use of sign-in sheets and telephone screeners

- Documenting of screen passes and failures, and patient visits
- Documenting of proper adherence to protocol windows
- Documenting of drug disposition
- Tracking of studies that are open, closed or pending
- Creating a system for records retention

Investigator Record Keeping

Disposition of the drug: An investigator is required to maintain adequate records of the disposition of the drug, including dates, quantity and use by subjects...

Case histories: An investigator is required to prepare and maintain adequate and accurate case histories that record all observations and other data pertinent to the investigation on each individual administered the investigational drug or employed as a control in the investigation. Case histories include the case report forms and supporting data including, for example, signed and dated consent forms and medical records including, for example, progress notes of the physician, the individual's hospital chart(s) and the nurse's notes. The case history for each individual shall document that informed consent was obtained prior to participation in the study.

Table 1 Source: 21 CFR Part 312.62

It is worth mentioning that the completion of paperwork is often considered to be a business function, not a medical function, yet the principal investigator, usually a physician, retains important responsibilities for study documentation. As detailed in Table 1, he or she is responsible for preparing and maintaining adequate records, tasks that cannot be given short shrift despite the investigator's many other responsibilities such as:[i]

- Ensuring that the investigation is conducted according to the signed FDA Statement of Investigator Form 1572
- Protecting the rights of human subjects
- Obtaining informed consent from each subject
- Controlling distribution of drugs, biologics or devices being investigated
- Assuring that an institutional review board (IRB) is provided information for initial and continuing review of the study

Telephone Screens, Sign-In Sheets, Universal Source Documents, etc.

Once the investigative site is initiated by the sponsor, the site is ready to begin the important steps of recruiting, enrolling and randomizing study subjects. This process generates its own slew of paperwork designed to document all patient interactions, including telephone screening, visits and all activities that occur at those visits. Operational control mechanisms include telephone screen sheets, scheduling logs, sign-in sheets, patient medical records, and case report forms (CRFs). Some of these documents belong in the regulatory binder, while others do not. The list of documents found in the regulatory binder appears in Chapter 4.

The necessary paperwork to screen and schedule pre-qualified candidates need not be complicated if proper forms have been developed and become part of the site's standard operating procedures (SOPs). Many of the documents are probably paper forms, but over time, more of them are likely to transition into electronic format.

The recruitment process begins with the initial call from a prospective patient, generally in response to an advertisement about the study or by physician referral. A designated phone screener answers the call and, using a prepared form that is typically computerized, collects basic demographic information from the caller. This screening form, and any scripts the recruiter uses, needs to be IRB-approved. It is crucial that the phone screener be cordial and professional so that the caller feels welcomed and valued. Small sites that are just starting to grow tend to have the study coordinator handle phone screening. But coordinators can quickly become too busy with study details to handle phone screening. A designated phone screener is the best person to field what can be lengthy telephone calls.

Once the demographic information is gathered, the screener asks a series of questions specific to the study about which the person is calling. Our experience at PBRC suggests that it is best to start with simple, innocuous questions, such as "Are you between the ages of 18 and 75?" The more sensitive questions, such as "Are you willing to prevent pregnancy while in the study?" are better left toward the end. The proper ordering of questions gives the phone screener an opportunity to develop a rapport with the caller so that interest and excitement about the study are more easily created.

If the patient passes the screen, he or she is referred to a scheduler to make an appointment. If the patient fails the phone screen, that person can be educated about other studies that are or will be recruiting and can be screened for those. To facilitate this process, a list of enrolling studies and the associated protocol screening sheets should be available to the screener. If the patient prequalifies for trials, he or she is referred to a scheduler for an appointment. In addition, the patient is asked about interest in having his or her information entered into the site's database. A sample screener appears in Table 2.

All screening calls are to be recorded in a log that is stored in the regulatory binder. Table 3 is a sample log.

Sample Telephone Screen

Name of study:
Name: Date:
Address:
City, State, Zip:
Phone (Home): Phone (Work):
Email:
DOB: Sex: Height: Weight:
Allergies:
Current Meds:
Medical/Surgical History:

1.	Are you between the ages of 18 and 75?	Yes	No	If no, patient is disqualified
2.	Do you have symptoms of reflux or heartburn at least twice per week?	Yes	No	If no, patient is disqualified
3.	Have you taken any of the following in the past 4 wks: Pepto Bismol, Prilosec, Prevacid (can take Axid, Zantac, Tagamet, Pepcid)	Yes	No	If yes, patient is disqualified
4.	Have you taken any of the following antibiotics in the past 4 wks: Cipro, Biaxin, Lorbid?	Yes	No	If yes, patient is disqualified
5.	Do you have known allergies to caprylic acid, citric acid or lauryl sulfate?	Yes	No	If yes, patient is disqualified
6.	Do you have any history within the last year of alcohol/drug dependence?	Yes	No	If yes, patient is disqualified
7.	Are you able to complete a (log) diary?	Yes	No	If no, patient is disqualified
8.	Are you willing to sign an informed consent form?	Yes	No	If no, patient is disqualified
9.	Can you take oral meds?	Yes	No	If no, patient is disqualified
10.	Are you willing to prevent pregnancy on this study?	Yes	No	If no, patient is disqualified

Referral Source: Screened by:

Table 2

Once a patient passes the telephone screen and comes to the site for a pre-qualifying physical exam or for any other purpose during the course of a study, he or she is to sign in on a sign-in sheet. This becomes one piece of evidence that the patient actually visited the site. Table 4 shows information to be included in the patient sign-in sheet and appointment book.

Sample Call Log

Date	Pt. Initials	Qualified for Study 123	Screen Failure–Reason	Referral Source
May 3	R.W.	Yes		Local paper
May 3	E.P.	No	Conflicting Med	Local radio
May 4	J.L.	Yes		PCP
May 4	S.L.	No	Hypertension	Local paper

Table 3

Information to Include in Patient Sign-in Sheets and the Appointment Book

Information to Include in Patient Sign-in Sheets and the Appointment Book
Date and time
Investigator's name
Study Coordinator's name
Study name
Visit number
Was appointment kept or canceled? If canceled, was appointment rescheduled?

Table 4

An overall review of the screening process appears in Figure 1.

Sample Screening Flow Chart

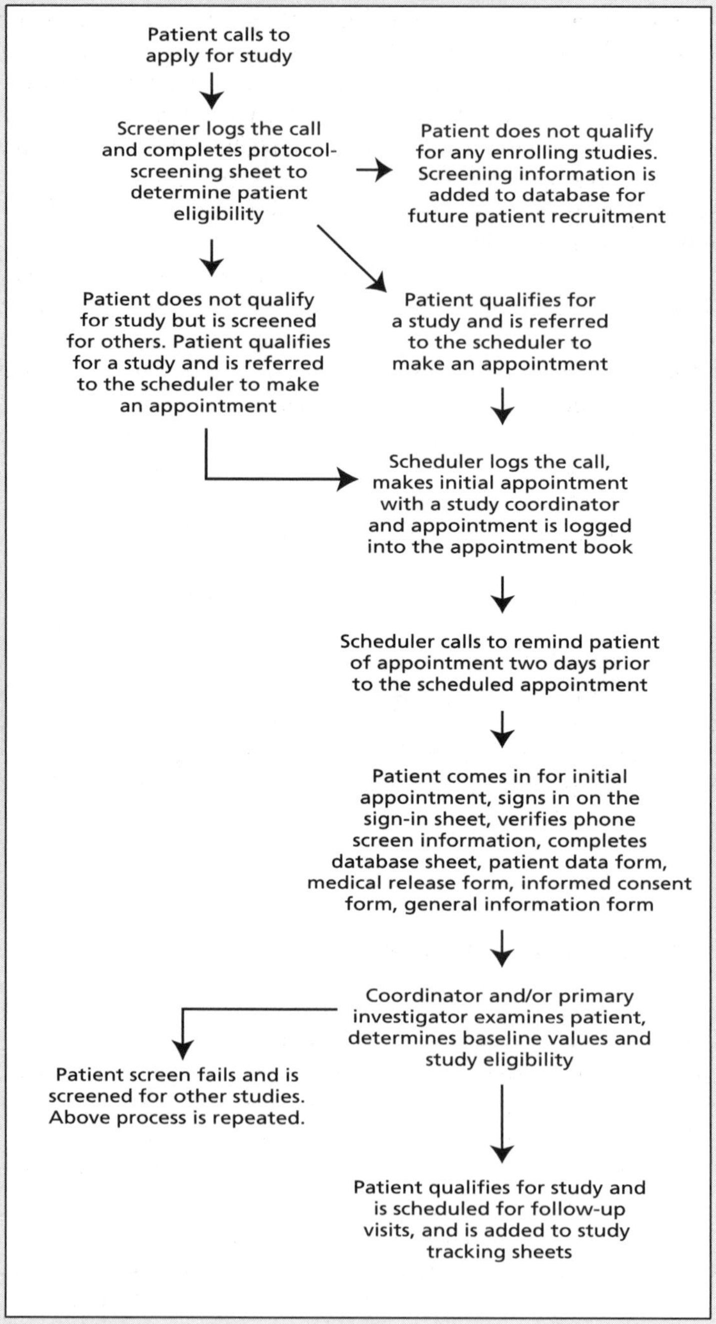

Patient calls to apply for study

↓

Screener logs the call and completes protocol-screening sheet to determine patient eligibility

→ Patient does not qualify for any enrolling studies. Screening information is added to database for future patient recruitment

↓ Patient does not qualify for study but is screened for others. Patient qualifies for a study and is referred to the scheduler to make an appointment

↘ Patient qualifies for a study and is referred to the scheduler to make an appointment

↓

Scheduler logs the call, makes initial appointment with a study coordinator and appointment is logged into the appointment book

↓

Scheduler calls to remind patient of appointment two days prior to the scheduled appointment

↓

Patient comes in for initial appointment, signs in on the sign-in sheet, verifies phone screen information, completes database sheet, patient data form, medical release form, informed consent form, general information form

↓

Coordinator and/or primary investigator examines patient, determines baseline values and study eligibility

← Patient screen fails and is screened for other studies. Above process is repeated.

↓

Patient qualifies for study and is scheduled for follow-up visits, and is added to study tracking sheets

Figure 1

The screening process can hit several bumps in the road. One of the most common is the "screen failure." This is a generic term that refers to patients who fail to qualify for a particular study at the time of the telephone screen. A screen failure is also defined as a patient who enrolls in a study but quickly exits from it because he or she no longer meets the inclusion/exclusion criteria. For example, a patient's laboratory values received by the site between the first and second visit may exclude the patient from continuing in the study. Whatever the source of the screen failure, the site must store the charts and source documents of those patients. In addition, the screening logs are to be kept that document patients who both pass and fail the preliminary telephone screen.[ii]

A quick word is in order regarding patients who screen fail following enrollment. These are patients who may have medical problems requiring resolution. They should be referred to a clinic or doctor's office for treatment. Setting up care for patients who screen fail can be a very positive experience both for the patient and the investigator. On occasion, a site may be able to persuade sponsors to provide medication on a compassionate use basis. Having the compassion to take this additional step may improve the patient's quality of life and creates good will. Also, it may lead to that patient both wanting to enroll in future studies and encouraging others to consider participating.

A case in point is the HIV patient who qualified for a study at a local site but opted not to participate because of the frequency of visits and the tests required. He was taking only herbal remedies, and no prescription medication. Through the help of a local organization and an infectious disease physician on staff at the site, antiviral medications were donated gratis to the patient. He was extremely grateful. He also started referring many people to the site and, despite his never having participated in a clinical trial, he remains the site's biggest fan.

Patient Records and Logs

Once the screening period is over, and the patient is officially enrolled and randomized, all of the steps composing the study must be documented. The growing site needs to establish forms, either paper or electronic, for this purpose. Some of the forms are complementary and validate each other. An example of a complementary system is the appointment book, the site sign-in sheet, and the tracking flow sheet. The appointment book shows the patient's appointment at a designated time. The sign-in sheet attests to the subject's appearance at the site at that designated appointment time, and the tracking flow sheet details the number of visits for the study and the activities and procedures to occur at each visit. For example, a chest x-ray is to occur on the second and fifth visits. After the patient has each x-ray, the scheduler notes that this procedure has occurred and records the date. The date for the procedure should match the date in the appointment book and on the patient sign-in sheet. The appointment book, sign-in sheet and tracking flow sheet serve as cross-checks within the system.

As noted in the budgeting chapter of this book, the tracking flow sheet can also be used for financial purposes. It is a useful tool both for developing costs for a study proposal, and for the signaling of invoices to be sent to the sponsor upon completion of procedures listed on the tracking sheet.

Some of the other necessary study tracking forms are listed below. Most of the forms listed below appear in Appendix c.

- **Patient Data** form—given to study volunteers to complete when they come in for the first study visit. This information is entered into the site database whether the patient eventually qualifies for the study or screen fails. The form is part of the initial study volunteer packet which includes a card naming the study, a questionnaire of medical history to be coded into the database and the items mentioned below.
- **Confidentiality** form—given to study volunteers when they register. This form states that study information is proprietary, so participants need to keep it confidential. In addition, the form says that patient records will be kept confidential and access to those records is limited to study staff on a need-to-know basis.
- **Medical Records Release** form—completed by patients indicating their willingness to have their medical records released to the site.
- **Medical Record Tracking** form—completed by the study coordinator when he or she receives medical records from the patient's doctor.
- **Forward Information to Physician** form—completed by a patient indicating whether he or she wants the data forwarded to the doctor.
- **Drug Dispensing** log—tracks who is taking study medication or placebo (maintaining blinding in non-open-label studies) and who is dispensing it. This form belongs in the regulatory binder.
- **Drug Transfer** log—tracks who takes the medication, how much each patient is taking and at which site the patient is taking it. It also tracks who is transporting the drug off-site, who has it and who is responsible for it. If the drug is returned to the site, then it is signed back in. This log is useful when using other doctors' offices or satellite sites.
- **Drug Disposition** log—keeps track of the number of pills returned to the sponsor at the end of a study and tallies what has been returned to the site by patients. It serves as a final inventory of the drugs in the study. This form belongs in the regulatory binder.
- **Laboratory Specimens** log—records when specimens are drawn, when they are shipped out, and when results are received and reviewed by the principal investigator. This form belongs in the regulatory binder.
- **Telephone** log—validates that certain phone calls were made during the study. It tracks calls made by the site to patients; made by patients

to the site; made by the monitor to the coordinator or principal investigator; made by the site to the monitor; or made by anyone during the course of the study. This log would also track emails between the site and the sponsor or CRO. These emails should be printed out and added to the log. This log belongs in the regulatory binder.

- **Visitor Sign-in** log—traces visits by monitors, sponsors or any other non-employee visits.
- A daily temperature chart for each refrigerator containing study-related items.
- Service logs for the photocopier, EKG machine and other equipment.

Tracking Patient Windows

When a patient misses or cancels an appointment, it must be re-scheduled within a required window of time. The site needs a reliable way to track these windows, a task that becomes more complex as the number of studies grows. If canceled appointments are not rescheduled within the required window, the patient may be disqualified from continued participation in a study.

The number of disqualified patients, or "dropouts," can be minimized through the use of a paper-based or basic software scheduling system designed to track therapeutic windows. Each study requires its own tracking timetable, a tool that needs to be set up at the beginning of each study. Included in the Appendix are tracking sheets that, if followed carefully, will ensure that no visits or procedures are missed.

To encourage the keeping of appointments, Palm Beach Research Center mails an "appointment reminder" card to patients seven days before each appointment. Also, a "next appointment" card is given to patients at each visit.

The establishment of good communication between the staff and patients starts with the very first contact and extends to all contacts with the patient. Showing the patient kindness and genuine interest tends to reduce the number of missed appointments. At the end of the study, we ask the patient to complete a "patient response" card, which provides us with feedback so that we can improve our systems, procedures and interactions with patients. By continuing to improve our operations, we aim to reduce the number of missed appointments.

Expand the Filing System and Plan for Record Retention and Storage

As the site grows, the number of patient charts and associated forms will escalate dramatically. To accommodate this expansion, the site needs to invest in a good filing system so that files from current studies are organized and easily accessible. Filing systems can be ordered from any number of medical supply vendors. Within the filing system, each patient should have one set of documents per trial. If that same patient enters into another trial at a later date, another set of documents should be created with a unique patient number to avoid possible mix-ups and to maintain patient confidentiality within each trial.

To minimize confusion among various ongoing studies, it is a good idea to purchase colored stickers so that each study can be color-coded. Placing the appropriately colored sticker on study boxes, bottles, patient files and forms for each study can reduce the chances of recording information for one study into a form belonging to another. As the industry slowly moves toward electronic reporting, the chance of doing this may be reduced if each form is accessed using a passcode specific to that study only.

When studies end, and as the number of documents mounts up, the site needs to arrange for off-site storage of older charts and records. It is preferable to have on-site storage because this setup allows ready access to the charts when needed for monitor, sponsor or FDA audits. In addition, easily accessed source documents from completed studies are excellent recruitment tools. Our experience at Palm Beach Research Center suggests that the best list of names to contact for a future study is the screen failure list from a similar study. Although an outpatient database is an important recruitment tool, certain studies require more specific criteria than are coded in our database. The more specific information is captured in screen failure lists and tends to yield better results when we use it to recruit for similar studies. For example, using this approach may allow us to do 40 or 50 targeted mailings instead of a mass mailing to thousands of names generated from our database.

Investigator Record Retention

An investigator shall retain records required to be maintained under this part for a period of 2 years following the date a marketing application is approved for the drug for the indication for which it is being investigated; or, if no application is to be filed or if the application is to be filed or if the application is not approved for such indication, until 2 years after the investigation is discontinued and FDA is notified.

Table 5 Source: 21 CFR Part 312.62

The reality is that a site is unlikely to have enough square footage to conform to federal storage requirements and to accommodate all of the documents continuously generated by an escalating number of trials. In the

United States, all study records must be stored for two years after the study drug is approved (Table 5). Sponsors often want investigators to retain their records for a period of five years after the study is completed. For international trials, storage requirements can extend to fifteen years.

Experienced clinical research associates (CRAs) recommend storing source documents along with the case report forms and regulatory binders, even though this requires more space and is costlier to maintain if the site is used to keeping regulatory binders at the site and the CRFs off-site. The CRA recommendation of storing both together also eliminates the problem that some sites create when they attempt to keep one source document for a patient regardless of how many studies he or she may participate in at the site. There should be one set of source documents created per patient per study.

Costs for moving records into and out of storage are a consideration and should be factored into study proposals. Sites that continue to absorb these costs will gradually see their profit margins decline.

We suggest that study records be reviewed for completeness prior to placing them in storage. A careful review will help to identify missing documents that may someday be required in future FDA or sponsor audits. We also recommend that patient records from a given study be stored either in alphabetical order or by randomization number, in which case a list is generated to cross-reference their names. Organizing the storage in this way will simplify recovery of needed charts. Taping or locking the boxes is recommended for added security. Although the storage facilities generally guarantee privacy, the information stored is confidential, so any extra precautions to safeguard the information is recommended.

When selecting a storage vendor, it is critical that the site choose one offering a secure and proper storage environment. Facilities that are wet or have poor quality storage boxes are to be avoided. The last thing an FDA inspector wants to hear is that the records were destroyed in a flood or were eaten by rodents.

Example 1 – The Sad Case of Improper Document Storage

An investigator in the Midwest owned a consistently high-enrolling site. His gross revenues from one particular sponsor exceeded $500,000 as a result of his conducting high quality studies that generated clean data. Several years ago, a Quality Assurance team from that sponsor conducted a routine audit of records from a study the investigator had completed the previous year. A few months prior to the audit, the investigator moved the records to the basement of his facility and placed them on the floor in piles. His motive in moving the records was to free up more space in his office.

This proved to be an unfortunate mistake. The records sustained water damage, which remained undetected until the QA team arrived. The records could have been salvaged had they been merely wet, but they had also been attacked by rodents who had eaten away most of the legible data, rendering them unsalvageable.

The situation was a tragedy for the sponsor and the investigator not to mention very embarrassing. When the records were removed from storage, they smelled of rodent droppings. The QA team departed without completing its investigation. Neither the QA team nor the sponsor ever returned to the site. The sponsor then tried to remove the investigator's data from its files, but later decided to repeat the trial without that investigator's participation.

As a result of this incident, the investigator started boxing his files appropriately. The cost to have prevented the water and rodent damage and maintain a relationship with the sponsor would have been $8.14, a typical annual cost to store one box at a storage facility.

Use Management Tools

Much of the discussion in this chapter addresses the various forms needed to document clinical activities at the site level. While most of the forms that are discussed exist today largely in paper format, management reports indicating site activity are more likely to have already transitioned to the computer. (See the "Electronic Medical Records and Other E-Solutions" chapter for more on this subject.)

For sites just expanding their clinical trials business, it is useful to select software designed to track several management activities related to patient and staff activities and allows networking among all computers at the site. In addition, the software should accommodate future growth by enabling the site to network with other sites. When shopping for software, consider packages that can create the following management tools (a sample of most of these forms is in Appendix c):

- **Study Synopsis** sheet—probably the most useful form for providing a quick overview of site activity. It tracks the status of all site studies and identifies the protocol number, PI, coordinator and back-up coordinator. The status of the study is noted by an "E" for enrolling, an "O" for over (completed) or "P" for pending. It notes the number of required vs. enrolled patients for each study. A sample is included in the Appendix.
- **Study Visit** report—tracks number of completed visits for each patient screened or enrolled in each trial. Patients are usually identified by patient number or by initials. The report should be able to provide a detailed breakdown of procedures completed at each visit for each patient that has been screened, enrolled and/or randomized. For example, it will show whether the patient has completed the informed consent, has had required physical examinations, laboratory tests, procedures, etc. Procedures and laboratory work that are not completed, or are completed but have not been recorded in the

case report forms, are identified. The report will also show if any of the visits were conducted outside of the designated window.

- **Adverse Event** report—tracks the study for any type of adverse events by the patient.
- **IRB** report—tracks IRB approvals as related to the study, i.e., approval of the protocol, approval of changes to the protocol and approval of informed consent form.

The above reports are for study-related functions. The software should also have business and budgeting capability. Our experience suggests that few programs on the market are designed for developing proposals and budgets for clinical trials, although this is changing. More vendors are designing software specific to the clinical trials industry. When considering use of a commercial package, it is important to test out the software on a trial basis. Another alternative is to hire a programmer to develop customized software for the site. If this route is chosen, the programmer should consider the fact that in the future, the site may need to network with other sites.

Some additional reports and logs related to business functions include:

- **Monthly Log of Number of Patients Randomized into Studies**—this log is valuable for tracking receivables if the site has contracts allowing for billing of enrollment milestones.
- **Monthly Study Timesheets for Study Coordinators**—this log allows the business manager to watch the coordinator costs for each study, and provides the site with benchmarks that can be used when calculating labor costs in bids for similar types of studies in the future.
- **Copy Request** form—helps the site track copying costs and charges for each study.
- **Forecast visits** report—forecasts study visits of enrolled patients. This report enables more efficient management of the site by noting when visits will be occurring so that study windows are met. For example, the report highlights if study visits are falling on a holiday or on a weekend, and facilitates appropriate rescheduling. Also, by noting when study visits are occurring, the site can keep better track of when to order needed supplies for required procedures.

The computer system should also be able to track:

- **Payments to all study subjects**
- **Visits from monitors, sponsors and federal auditors**—this log will verify that visits noted on the case report forms did, in fact, occur.

Use Office Equipment to Grow the Site

As a site grows and more studies are added, the need for office efficiency becomes increasingly important. High-speed copiers are essential to copy protocols quickly. Multiple fax lines are needed to keep the flow of information moving among sponsors, CROs and the site. A postal machine is invaluable in sending out large numbers of mailings and keeping track of mailing costs. An upgraded telephone system offering voice mail and conference calling capability is a must. A desktop or laptop computer dedicated to correspondence avoids a situation in which a study coordinator needs to enter study data on a computer, while another staff member needs to use that same computer to send out follow-up correspondence that must go out by 5:00 PM.

An investment in basic office equipment may seem costly initially, but it will save the site many people-hours. Just as important, proper equipment will create a professional image for the site. Poor-quality photocopies or outdated phone systems make the site seem less than serious about the business of clinical trials.

Example – Project a Professional Image

I will be eternally grateful to the first study broker with whom I worked. When I first started doing trials, I was anxious to do more. John, a broker, was recommended to me as someone who had previously worked for one of the larger sponsors and had developed a good reputation and many contacts. I met John and was impressed with the extent of his contacts in the industry and by the fact that he was articulate and knowledgeable.

Following our meeting, I sent John a thank-you letter, stating our interest in working with him to procure more trials. He sent me a return letter that taught me an invaluable lesson in research and in life. He had photocopied my letter and noted two spelling errors. My secretary and I had both neglected to proofread the letter. John's point and lesson was: How could a sponsor trust our site to produce clean, accurate data when we couldn't even produce a simple correspondence without spelling errors? John refused to work with us after this incident. Now, not a letter, CRF or any other document ever leaves our site without careful proofreading. I have been grateful to him ever since.

In Review

The site's growing process requires the implementation of many forms and logs to document and track all the steps taken to complete a clinical study. Many of the forms, such as the screening log, drug dispensing log and the laboratory specimen log belong in the regulatory binder. These are the forms that document ethical conduct of the study. There is also a need for the site to use business forms that function as management tools. A few of these are the study synopsis sheet and the monthly log of the number of patients randomized into studies. These logs and others track the financial status of the site as a function of enrollment and signal when a site needs to generate invoices to sponsors.

Finally, as the site is implementing its array of study and financial tracking forms, there needs to be an investment in professional office equipment such as high-speed copiers, postage machines and enough computers to make the site function as an efficient, well-managed business.

References

[i] Title 21 Code of Federal Regulations (CFR) 50, 312, 812.

[ii] Title 21 Code of Federal Regulations (CFR) 312.62, "Investigator record keeping and record retention."

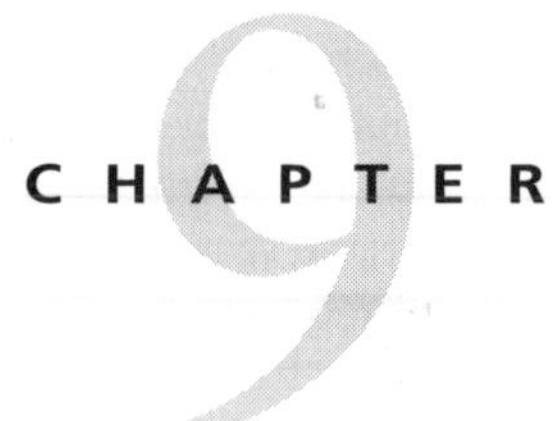

CHAPTER 9

Electronic Medical Records and Other E-Solutions

- What Is an Electronic Medical Record (EMR)?
- What Electronic Medical Records Mean to the Investigative Site
- The Impact of HIPAA on the EMR Market
- Beyond EMRs
- A Look at Web-Based Clinical Trials
- 21 CFR Part 11–Legislation Enabling Electronic Records and Electronic Signatures
- In Review

Throughout this book, I make frequent reference to the need for extensive documentation during the entire clinical trials process. Every step along the drug development path must be recorded, starting with pre-trial submissions to the institutional review board (IRB), moving to informed consent activities, patient visit procedures, data collection and submission, and ending with study close-out. And all of these documents must be properly maintained and retained for two years after a study drug is either approved or its investigation is discontinued and the FDA is notified.[i] Because of these requirements, sites must have appropriate on-site storage capability plus additional off-site storage.

The need for storage capability is bound to continue for some time because research suggests that less than 5% of today's patient charts, for example, exist in electronic form.[ii] They, like most source documents and other trial-related forms, are still overwhelmingly completed with pen and paper. This low-tech approach in an otherwise high-tech industry reflects the fact that the pharmaceutical industry is notoriously behind the curve in adopting technologies to improve clinical development processes. It has been reported that the information technology expenditures of the pharmaceutical industry are approximately 4% to 6% of company sales—half of the 8% to 10% of sales spent by companies in other information-intensive industries.[iii]

Things are slowly changing, however. Electronic medical record (EMR) systems now exist that allow physicians to: [iv,v]

- Document patient visits according to HCFA guidelines using wireless, handheld personal digital assistant (PDA), touch screen and voice technology
- Analyze patient population of the practice by disease and demographics
- Access chart information from the Internet and private servers
- Store charts in an encrypted form in a secured data center
- Pull the chart to a computer to add more notes
- Allow paper copies to be printed out

EMR systems offering these electronic features are promising in many ways. Using wireless tablet or handheld technologies, EMRs enable the direct input of data into electronic patient charts at the point of care, a step that could reduce errors linked to repetitive data entry, data transcription, illegible handwriting or omission. Also, the electronic format allows analysis and searching of the patient database, activities that are useful for patient recruitment purposes. There is the convenience of controlled Internet access to medical records needed by physicians working in satellite locations. Finally, use of EMRs can reduce the tremendous storage and maintenance burden created by a paper-driven industry.

In 2000, the Medical Records Institute, a global healthcare informatics forum, conducted a multi-question survey of more than 500 physicians, chief information officers, medical information systems analysts, company presidents, network managers and others to determine the usage trends of electronic health records. When asked, "What are the major clinical factors that are driving the need for electronic health record systems," the key reasons given by 296 respondents were:[vi]

- Improve the ability to share patient record information among healthcare providers – 85%
- Improve clinical processes or workflow efficiency – 81%
- Improve quality of care – 80%
- Provide access to patient records at remote locations – 71%
- Improve clinical data capture – 68%

Even with the promise of so many benefits, the adoption rate of EMRs remains slow. In that same survey, the Medical Records Institute identified major barriers to implementing electronic health records. Responses appear in Table 1.

Major Barriers to Plans for Implementing an Electronic Health Record (n=286)

Reason	Percentage
Lack of adequate funding or resources	57%
Difficulty in justifying the investment	40%
Inability to find a vendor or technical solution that addresses the needs of "my organization"	36%
Difficulty in implementing an information solution in a rapidly changing environment	34%
Inadequate or incomplete healthcare information standards, data sets or code sets	31%
Lack of nationally accepted guidelines and policies to protect the confidentiality of health records	28%
Difficulty in creating a migration plan from paper to electronic health records	27%
Lack of support by medical staff	27%
Lack of consensus to commit to specific vendor or technical solution	20%
Lack of support by the executive hierarchy	19%
Other	6%

Table 1 Source: www.medrecinst.com

In an unrelated research effort, the American Medical Association (AMA) pointed to "lack of standards" as one of the biggest barriers to acceptance of healthcare information technology.[vii] To address this issue, the AMA's Council on Medical Services devised a survey tool that it circulated to twenty-nine external advisors to gather a comprehensive listing of data elements to be included in an optimal EMR system. The Council believes that the results of this survey could provide standards to EMR vendors to help them optimize the usefulness of their products.[viii] The acceptance of standardized data elements by physicians can fuel the market for electronic medical records, which has an estimated potential of $3 billion in gross revenues by 2005.[ix]

What Is an Electronic Medical Record (EMR)?

An electronic medical record is "an upgraded version of the computerized medical record that has essentially the same structure, scope and information as the paper-based record; however, the information is re-arranged for computer use. The EMR should also be capable of appropriately capturing, processing and storing information and be inter-operable with other related systems such as billing and administration."[x]

The electronic medical record is a more evolved form of the computerized medical record, which generally resides wholly within a desktop or intranet server that can accept input or scanned data from paper. Unlike the EMR, computerized medical records generally use document imaging technology. They are not interactive and, typically, data contained within them are not configured to contribute to databases scattered among various systems.[xi]

While EMRs seem to have reached only a small share of their market potential, the computer-based patient record is taking root in healthcare facilities of various sizes as well as physician group practices. Results of a 2001 survey conducted by the Healthcare Information and Management Systems Society (HIMSS) revealed that 29% of 532 respondents report working in institutions that have begun to install computerized patient record hardware and software (Figure 1).[xii] Survey respondents mostly represent information technology management at healthcare facilities. The survey asked specifically about the status of "computer-based patient records" at their facilities, and did not ask respondents to differentiate between that term and "electronic patient records." Although it is possible that respondents interpreted the two terms interchangeably, it is more likely that they answered the question in reference to computerized patient records, and not EMRs, because today's customers are opting more for EMRs that reside on intranet servers that they control within the confines of a specific institution or group of affiliated institutions.[xiii]

What Electronic Medical Records Mean to the Investigative Site

In an ideal scenario, a site would collect and transmit source data, make entries into patient records and make required IRB submissions, all electronically. Although the typical site is not yet operating this way, it may be in the not-too-distant future. Some in the industry believe that once a few key players set the standard by implementing system-wide electronic solutions, there will be an industry-wide stampede to jump aboard.[xiv]

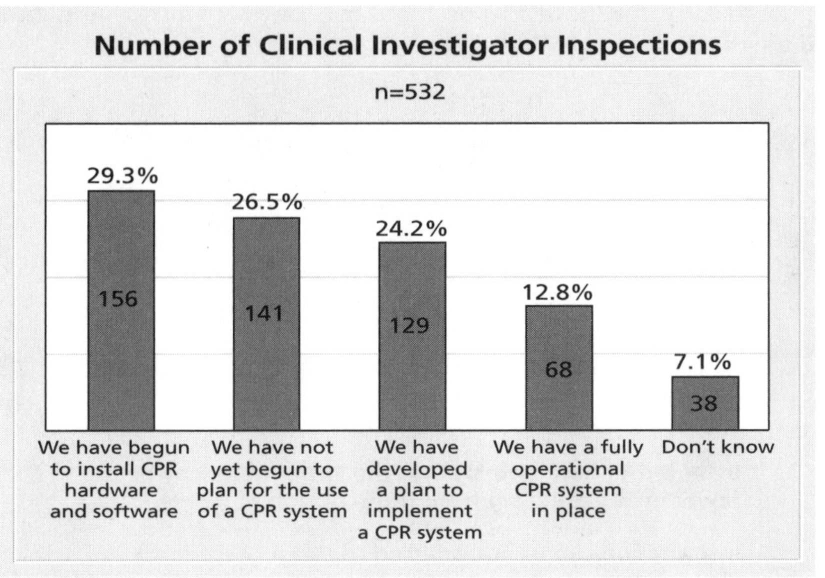

Figure 1 Source: www.himss.org, 2001

When EMRs are in place at the site, they will serve several key functions (Table 2). One of the most critical is that investigators can use them for patient recruitment purposes as the patients' diagnoses, laboratory results, scans, hospital and pharmacy information will be available in a screenable database format. For example, if a study is seeking controlled non-insulin-dependent diabetic patients with hypertension and normal serum creatinine, a search of an EMR database can possibly identify patients who meet these criteria within minutes. This happens simply by typing the criteria into the EMR query system. Harvesting this information from a system of paper records could take weeks or months.

In addition, EMRs accessed via a handheld device, such as a personal digital assistant (PDA), could be used to flag potential study patients during office visits. For example, as the doctor enters data during a patient visit, if that profile happens to match selection criteria for a trial, information about that trial will appear, reminding the physician to discuss it with the patient.[xv]

One of today's more difficult challenges for EMRs is that they may not be able to supply all of the necessary information into electronic case report forms. If, for example, the case report form asks if the patient has had any gastrointestinal symptoms within the past two months, a computerized EMR system may not be able to determine that a patient who experienced diarrhea last month could be considered to have had a gastrointestinal episode. For this reason, there may still need to be some degree of human review of patient records while EMR systems become more integrated into the clinical trials process.[xvi] Despite this issue, the power of EMR systems is not diminished because the patients whose data are reviewed by humans prior to entry into the case report forms may have been quickly identified during a search of an EMR database.

How the Site Can Benefit by Using Electronic Medical Records (EMRs)

Recruitment purposes: 1. Search database of EMRs quickly using inclusion/exclusion criteria 2. With EMRs on a personal digital assistant, physician can be reminded to discuss trials with patient for which he or she may qualify.
By entering data directly into the EMR, there may be fewer errors resulting from transcription mistakes.
Information can be transmitted to the sponsor or CRO via the Internet, using highly secured access.
Paper burden is reduced.

Table 2

The Impact of HIPAA on the EMR Market

If you are unfamiliar with HIPAA, you will learn about it once your investigative site considers implementing an EMR system. HIPAA refers to the Health Insurance Portability and Accountability Act of 1996 (Public Law 104-191). It is a broad-based federal law signed by President Clinton on August 21, 1996. Its purpose is to improve the efficiency and effectiveness of the healthcare system by encouraging the development of healthcare information systems using electronic data interchange (EDI) for health-related administrative and financial transactions.[xvii] In addition, HIPAA seeks to establish the required use of national transaction standards while maintaining patient privacy when business and patient information is transmitted electronically between organizations. HIPAA compliance will be a major effort estimated to cost two to three times as much as Y2K initiatives for the entire healthcare industry.[xviii]

The Administrative Simplification component of HIPAA requires the Department of Health and Human Services (HHS) to develop standards and requirements for maintenance and transmission of health information that identifies individual patients. This component contains sections that will directly influence efforts to bring electronic solutions, such as EMRs, to the conduct of clinical trials. All vendors of EMR systems must conform to the standards in the Administrative Simplification component.

This component encompasses four standards:

1. Electronic transactions and code sets
2. Privacy of individually identifiable health information
3. Security to preserve patient confidentiality
4. Creation of unique health identifiers for patients, health plans, providers and employers

Final regulations for the first standard were published by the HHS on August 17, 2000, and went into effect sixty days later. This spawned a twenty-four-month period for healthcare clearinghouses, healthcare providers and large health plans to come into compliance. At that time, October 16, 2002, they will be required to have implemented systems to accept standardized financial and administrative data via EDI.

Alternatively, compliance can be delayed by one year as a result of a bill signed by President Bush on December 7, 2001. This action enables entities covered by HIPAA to delay compliance until October 16, 2003. To qualify for the extra year, entities must submit a compliance plan to the Secretary of the HHS by October 16, 2002. The compliance plan must include a budget schedule, work plan and implementation strategy for achieving compliance.

Final privacy regulations (Standard 2) were published at the end of December 2000, during the last days of the Clinton administration, and were implemented by the George W. Bush administration on April 14, 2001. Healthcare clearinghouses, healthcare providers and large health plans have until April 14, 2003, to come into compliance, whereas smaller health plans have an additional year. By the April 2003 implementation deadline, a few changes to the final privacy regulations are anticipated, which are expected to be worked into the final document. Security regulations (Standard 3) may be developed next.

The fourth standard is one part of HIPAA that will directly affect clinical research. It addresses standards by which unique patient-identifying information can be transmitted electronically, possibly over the Internet.

With growing concern over privacy issues, there is a great deal of interest in unique health identifiers for patients. Although they will use encryption, they will identify specific individuals. Investigative sites do not send names of study volunteers to sponsors or CROs, but there is still enough confidential information to require encryption. As of this writing, HHS has not yet published patient-identifying regulations. Regulations have been proposed for unique identifiers for national providers and employers, but they have not been finalized as of this writing.

The patient-identifying standard notwithstanding, development of standards through HIPAA is generally viewed as enabling to the adoption of EMRs because lack of standards is considered to be a major stumbling block in their acceptance. Standardized data elements used by all vendors and providers will go a long way toward growing the e-environment.

Beyond EMRs

In addition to EMRs, other types of e-solutions are emerging to streamline data collection at the site level. The promise of electronic solutions is the speeding of data collection while reducing both the number of errors and the paper burden. Fewer mistakes in data gathering should lead to a shortened time needed for data collection and management, a process that currently accounts for as much as two-thirds of clinical trial cycle time (Figure 2).

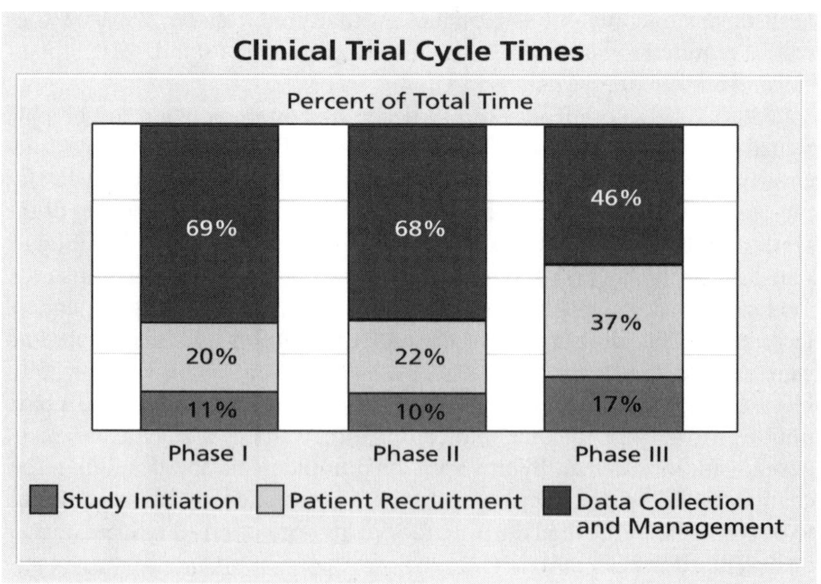

Figure 2 Source: CenterWatch

Besides EMRs, other parts of the clinical trial that are destined for increased use of electronic solutions are:

- Electronic case report forms (eCRFs)
- Web-enabled electronic data capture (EDC)
- Patient recruitment via the Internet
- Electronic signatures
- Electronic patient diaries
- Electronic submission of regulatory documents

Electronic data capture (EDC), which is now on the radar screen, refers to the process of collection of data into a persistent electronic form (i.e., modem-based, web-based, pen-based,* fax-based and interactive voice-response data collection applications).[xix] Using EDC, information can be entered into an electronic case report form (eCRF), which may become the source document. The eCRF can exist on a desktop computer, a laptop, possibly a handheld personal digital assistant (PDA) or on an electronic tablet. Each has advantages and disadvantages in terms of portability and ease of data entry. Some eCRFs may require the investigator to type information into specific data fields. Others may be formatted using a template, and the investigator selects the appropriate choice with an electronic pen.

Today, it is generally acknowledged that physicians are unlikely to type information into electronic forms in the presence of patients either because they lack typing skills or more importantly, because they view the entering of data as obtrusive and disruptive to the doctor-patient relationship. Being careful to enter data correctly into an electronic device turns the investigator's attention away from the patient and toward the device. This problem does not exist with old-fashioned paper and pen because the doctor can scribble notes rather inconspicuously while talking to or examining the patient. For this reason and others, some sites may opt to retain the paper case report form as the original source document, and then later transcribe the notes into an electronically formatted CRF. Retaining the paper CRF means that there is still a step requiring a human to review the entering of data. This is someone who can spot misspelled words or the writing of a wrong date, and make that correction before entering the data into the electronic system.

Additional reasons for maintaining the paper CRF source document stem from the fact that e-solutions are so new that it is not always clear how to implement electronic source documents without violating good clinical practice (GCP). Source documents, for example, must be attributable to the individual who created them. One way to do this is for an individual to create a paper CRF as the source document and then transcribe the data into an electronic source, such as a computer. The site maintains control of this paper CRF source document. Once the transition is made to using the eCRF as the source document, the computer on which it was created must remain

* "Pen-based" refers to systems that use a pen to collect information electronically, such as the type used with a personal digital appliance (PDA).

in the control of the investigator or institution along with system controls and operating procedures to guarantee that the data are not changed or manipulated.[xx] The next step is for the eCRF to be created on a web server-based system, whereby data are stored directly on a server, generally at the sponsor's or CRO's facility, rather than at the investigative site. Because these data are not stored under the direct control of the investigator, it could potentially violate a GCP rule that source documents must be stored under the control of the site.[xxi]

The introduction of handheld PDAs into the clinical data collection process also raises issues about control of source data. Wireless PDAs can be formatted to produce an electronic CRF. If that eCRF contains the primary source data, the site must maintain control of the archival copy and must be able to retrieve it. The challenge is that PDAs are typically battery powered, and if that battery is removed and the memory lost within a few minutes of battery removal, a question arises as to whether PDAs offer the kind of storage that is defined as permanent or archival. PDAs generally offer flash memory or backup memory that allows the device to persist without power from the main battery. Although the data can be transferred to a hard disk for storage, a medium that is considered to be durable, is the PDA considered to house the source document?

According to comments by FDA officials, if the PDA can record data in a manner that can be saved and retrieved, it is considered to house source data, making it subject to the same record retention guidelines that apply to paper-driven trials (Table 3).[xxii] This position suggests that the agency is re-examining its original thinking on the subject of "durable media."[xxiii] Although an FDA publication, *Guidance for Industry, Computerized Systems Used in Clinical Trials*, states "A record is created when it is saved to durable media,"[xxiv] there is no clear definition of "durable media."

"Computerized systems should ensure that all applicable regulatory requirements for record keeping and records retention in clinical trials are met with at least the same degree of confidence as is provided with paper systems."

Table 3 Source: Computers in Clinical Trials Draft Guidance–Implications, 6/24/97

Recently, the FDA began exploring a broader interpretation of "durable media" as a result of the expanded use of devices with transient memory and the passage of the Electronic Signatures in Global and National Commerce Act. This act, which was signed into law by President Clinton in June 2000, very broadly defines an electronic record as "information that is inscribed on a tangible medium or that is stored in an electronic or other medium and is retrievable in perceivable form."[xxv] No mention is made of the transience or permanence of storage technology.

At this point in time, much of the discussion about durable media is rather academic because the number of sites using PDA technology, electronic tablets, laptops or desktop computers for EDC is believed to be small. There are no definitive data attesting to this, but a recent survey of 229 clinical research professionals (mostly study coordinators and monitors) suggests that use of EDC is indeed limited. Although 49% reported that their companies had used EDC systems at some point in time, more than 80% reported that no trials were currently being conducted at their sites using EDC.[xxvi]

As more and more sites start participating in EDC trials, they need to establish standard operating procedures (SOPs) that describe how to implement electronic data collection systems. The SOPs should address system setup and installation, data collection, system maintenance, data backup and recovery, security and change control.[xxvii]

A Look at Web-Based Clinical Trials

As major pharmaceutical sponsors seek ways to reduce the clinical development timeline for their investigational products, they are undoubtedly investing in web-enabled initiatives. A secured network, operating among multiple sites, the CRO and the sponsor, should speed data transmission, improve data quality and eliminate problems inherent in storing source data in a specific site-based computer that is running a local application, must have frequent backups and must be locked up.

Currently, there are two scenarios. First is a pure Internet browser-based application that operates in online mode with local web browsers, without additional software. Data can be transmitted to a central database in real time, queries can be handled more quickly and the data are cleaner, earlier.[xxviii] The second option may be more commonplace today and may be an intermediate step on the way to pure Internet-based trials. This choice offers a mix of offline data entry (but still electronic) using specialized local applications, followed by sending the data via the Internet at a later time.

There are reasons why this hybrid approach can be useful. Some sites may have slow Internet connections, which can make data entry and transmission slow and frustrating. Also, by using a hybrid system, people can enter data off-line from any laptop, PDA or electronic tablet associated with the study. This means they can enter data at home, in the evenings and on weekends, and then upload later from a secured line at the site when it is convenient. Additional reasons for continuing with a hybrid system appear in Table 4.

As more trial data start moving toward web-based transmission, bandwidth becomes an issue. Bandwidth refers to the transmission capacity of a network medium and is measured in bits per second. The more information to be sent in a given period of time, the more bandwidth is required. Without appropriate bandwidth, data transmission can become slow and tedious. For this reason, vendors offering e-solutions to clinical trials can best improve the speed of web-based data transmission by developing small page sizes, using limited bits of information and graphics. This enables sites with slower dial-up Internet connections to download and upload pages more quickly. This convenience factor will go a long way toward speeding adoption of this technology.

Reasons for Continuing with a Hybrid Offline-Online EDC System
Some sites may have slow Internet connections, which can make data entry frustrating.
Entering data offline can add an element of convenience allowing data to be entered into a laptop, for instance, and then later uploaded.
Some rural sites and locations outside the U.S. may have weak Internet infrastructures.
Some studies that are hospital-based may occur in rooms, i.e., operating rooms, that may lack Internet access.
Some sites have computers with operating systems that have limited database tools and lack sufficient security features for pure Internet-based trials.

Table 4 Source: Contract Pharma, June 2001

21CFR Part 11 – Legislation Enabling Electronic Records and Electronic Signatures

On August 20, 1997, FDA regulations, known as 21CFR Part 11 of the Code of Federal Regulations, went into effect. A revised version took effect on April 1, 2000. These regulations provide criteria under which the Food and Drug Administration (FDA) will accept electronic records and electronic signatures that it considers to be equal to handwritten paper documents and signatures. It is this set of regulations that allows clinicians to record a first observation electronically and ultimately enables sponsors to make electronic submissions[xxix] (Table 5).

Part 11 regulations are destined to have profound impact. As sponsors start taking advantage of electronic submissions, and sites begin recording first observations electronically, the mountains of paper will start to diminish, along with the number of errors associated with completing, transcribing and maintaining complex paper records. Yet, as with all new technology, there must be a way to assure it is as reliability as the old, familiar method, which in this case is paper documentation. First, each configuration of hardware and software must be validated to ensure accuracy, reliability, consistent intended performance and the ability to discern invalid or altered records. Validation of a system refers to documented evidence that the system does what it purports to do and will continue to do so over the life of the system.[xxx] Secondly, an electronic system must be able to generate accurate and complete copies of all documents. Some of the other requirements appear in Table 6.

Sec. 11.1 (a) "The regulations in this part set forth the criteria under which the agency considers electronic records, electronic signatures and handwritten signatures executed to electronic records to be trustworthy, reliable, and generally equivalent to paper records and handwritten signatures executed on paper."

Sec. 11.1 (b) "This part applies to records in electronic form that are created, modified, maintained, archived, retrieved or transmitted, under any records requirements set forth in agency regulations...."

Table 5 Source: 21 CFR Part 11 Subpart A—General Provisions

In Review

For an investigative site that is aiming to grow, accommodating the storage needs for an ever increasing number of paper medical records and all of the associated study source documentation can become quite burdensome. Not only do good clinical practice guidelines require that the study documents be stored for a period of two years after the study ends, they must be stored in a way that will maintain them in good condition.

By introducing electronic solutions, sites stand to gain many benefits. Electronic medical records (EMRs) can shrink the paper mountains substantially. They offer other useful features as well such as the ability to enter data directly into EMRs, eliminating the step of writing first on paper and then transcribing the information into the chart. Perhaps the most useful aspect of EMRs is that they can become powerful patient recruitment tools as data housed within the charts are searchable, enabling sites to identify

Some Electronic Records System Requirements per 21 CFR Part 11
Validation
Ability to generate accurate and complete copies of records in both human readable and electronic form
Archival protection of records
Audit trails
System controls
Personnel training and qualifications
Establishment of and adherence to written policies that hold individuals accountable and responsible for actions initiated under their electronic signatures
System, controls and documentation are subject to inspection

Table 6 Source: 21 CFR Part 11

potential study subjects much more quickly than by using traditional methods of reviewing paper charts coupled with costly, broad-based patient recruitment campaigns.

Adding to the menu of e-solutions are technologies for electronic data capture and transmission, electronic patient diaries and electronic submissions to institutional review boards. The idea of these e-solutions is to improve the quality and speed of data collection. This should reduce the amount of time that the sponsor spends on data cleaning, an activity that utilizes nearly 32% of the clinical development timeline.

In an effort to move toward paperless clinical trials, challenges remain. If source data are to be captured during a patient visit, the physician must enter the first observation directly into an electronic medical record of electronic data capture form. This means that he or she is either typing into a computer or electronic tablet or selecting choices on a handheld device. In either case, this activity turns the physician's attention away from the patient and toward the device. It is also worth mentioning that it is generally recognized that physicians are highly unlikely to type information into an electronic format in front of the patient. Because of this obstacle and other issues, some users of electronic products continue to collect that first observation on paper, and later transcribe the data into an electronic format.

Despite these glitches, electronic clinical trials are here to stay. It is believed that virtually every major sponsor has an ongoing electronic data capture initiative.[xxxi] Also, federal regulations in the form of HIPAA and 21CFR Part 11 are seen as enablers or facilitators of electronic clinical trials. They serve to standardize data collection, an element that is considered essential to adoption of electronic technology, and they address critical issues of privacy, such as encryption.

Moving from paper-based trials to electronic clinical trials is now evolving. It is possible that once a few major vendors implement successful end-to-end electronic solutions, others will jump on the bandwagon.

References

[i] 21 Code of Federal Regulations (CFR) Part 312.62.

[ii] US Bancorp Piper Jaffray, 2001.

[iii] "Get Ready for eR&D," *R&D Directions*, R&D Staff, Nov./Dec. 1999, p. 68.

[iv] *www.medicalogic.com/products/logician_internet/overview/chart room_overview.html*, accessed June 8, 2001.

[v] *www.powermed.com/powermed_features.htm*, accessed June 8, 2001.

[vi] *www.medrecinst.com*, accessed June 8, 2001.

[vii] *www.ama-assn.org/ama/pub/category/2903.html*, accessed June 11, 2001.

[viii] *www.ama-assn.org/ama/pub/category/2912.html*, accessed June 11, 2001.

[ix] US Bancorp Piper Jaffray, 2001.

[x] *www.medrecinst.com*, accessed February 25, 2001.

[xi] Ibid.

[xii] *www.himss.org/2001survey/nonvender/pages/results27.htm.*, accessed June 12, 2001.

[xiii] Discussion with Mark Leavitt, M.D., Ph.D., MedScape, Inc., June 22, 2001. Information provided by HIMSS public relations spokesperson (June 12, 2001).

[xiv] "Clinical Research in Transition, 2001 ACRP White Paper," *The Monitor*, Jim Maloy et al., Summer 2001, Vol. 15, Issue 2, p. 20.

[xv] Ibid., "Clinical Research in Transition, 2001 ACRP White Paper," p. 23.

[xvi] Discussion with Mark Leavitt, M.D., Ph.D., MedScape, Inc., June 22, 2001.

[xvii] *http://www.smed.com/hipaa/overview.php*, accessed June 14, 2001.

[xviii] "Health-Care Industry Faces Task That May Rival Y2K," *The Wall Street Journal*, Carol Gentry, January 3, 2000, p. 3.

[xix] Clinical Data Interchange Standards Consortium (CDISC), *www.cdisc.org*.

[xx] According to Jim McCormick, Ph.D., of the FDA's Division of Compliance Policy in the Office of Enforcement, 21 Code of Federal Regulations (CFR) Part 11 does allow investigators to migrate to more contemporary electronic applications as long as information is

not lost and the knowledge that is conveyed in the original record is migrated to the new system. This conversation took place on June 29, 2001.

[xxi] "e-source; To e or not to e," *Applied Clinical Trials*, Paul Bleicher, May 2001, p. 2.

[xxii] Ibid., *Applied Clinical Trials*, p. 2.

[xxiii] John C. McKenney, SEC Associates, Inc., *Update on the "Durable Media" Debate*, November 20, 2000.

[xxiv] Guidance for Industry, Computerized Systems Used in Clinical Trials, Section 5.B.1.a, *www.fda.gov/ora/compliance_ref/bimo/ffinalcct.pdf.*

[xxv] Electronic Signatures in Global and National Commerce Act, Public Law 106-229, Sec. 106 (9).

[xxvi] "Electronic Data Capture: Survey 2000," *The Monitor*, Renita E. Feller, BLS, Spring 2001, pp. 38-39.

[xxvii] *Computers in Clinical Trials, Draft Guidance, Implications*, July 17, 1997, *www.fda.gov/cder*, accessed June 25, 2001.

[xxviii] "Making the Move to Web-Based Clinical Trials," *Contract Pharma*, Paul Bleicher, June 2001, pp. 36-38.

[xxix] "Clinical Research in Transition, 2001 ACRP White Paper," *The Monitor*, Jim Maloy et al., Summer 2001, Vol. 15, Issue 2, p. 21.

[xxx] *www.phaseforward.com*, accessed June 25, 2001.

[xxxi] "Clinical Research in Transition, 2001 ACRP White Paper," *The Monitor*, Jim Maloy et al., Summer 2001, Vol. 15, Issue 2, p. 19.

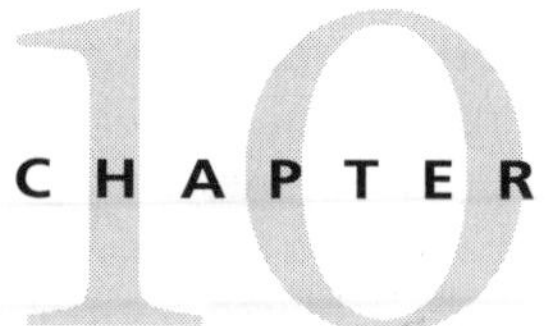

Patient Recruitment and Enrollment – Critical to Success

- The Nuts and Bolts of a Multi-Dimensional Patient Recruitment Campaign
- National Recruitment Campaigns
- Newer Methods of Recruiting
- Metrics
- The Clinical Trial Volunteer
- Patient Retention
- In Review

An investigative site's very survival depends upon its ability to recruit and enroll the contracted number of study subjects. As technological advances lead to pipelines rich with new chemical entities, sponsors need to identify subjects willing and able to enroll in and complete the resulting clinical trials, currently numbering between 50,000 and 60,000 annually in the United States.[i,ii] At present, nearly 4,400 patients are needed per new drug application (NDA), a figure that has jumped 23% since the early 1990s[iii] (Figure 1).

Data suggest that many more patients are needed, not only to fill ongoing and projected studies, but also to offset the poor patient retention rate. Of the estimated 3 million people who start the clinical trials process annually for industry-sponsored trials, only 700,000 complete those studies.[iv] The dropout rate is high for many reasons: the study subject who comes in for the screening visit does not qualify; the subject loses interest; the subject is unreliable; the subject moves away; the subject experiences an adverse reaction. At present, for every twenty patients who respond to a patient recruitment solicitation or referral, only one will complete a clinical trial.[v] These odds highlight the difficulty inherent in recruiting, enrolling and retaining study subjects. In fact, recruitment and enrollment activities consume 22.3% of the clinical development timeline.[vi] Assuming clinical drug trials in the United States cost $8 billion annually, the patient enrollment piece translates into a yearly expenditure of $1.78 billion.[vii]

Despite this huge sum, lagging recruitment is the largest cause of lost time in clinical trials. One study showed that almost 80% of all clinical trials must extend their enrollment periods by at least one month.[viii] Another study of 400 sites revealed that 86% of phase II and phase III clinical trials failed to recruit study subjects within the contracted enrollment period. This study also showed that the recruitment period for the typical trial is extended an average of two months.[ix]

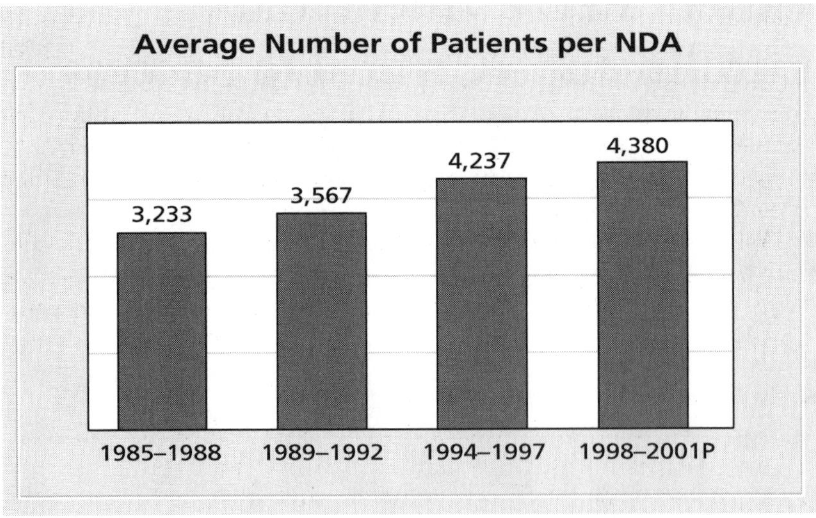

Figure 1 Source: Tufts, CSDD, 1999; Peck, C., Food and Drug Law Journal 1997

As sponsors continue outsourcing study conduct activities, the heavy responsibility of patient enrollment is falling squarely on the investigative site. How the site fares with these responsibilities can spell the difference between success and just barely making it. A site that promises to enroll twenty patients for a study within the specified recruitment period but ends up with only three or four enrollees will probably damage its credibility with that sponsor, particularly for future studies in that therapeutic area.

Fortunately, since the mid-1990s, many sponsors have acknowledged that various methods are often needed to recruit patients in a timely fashion, and they are willing to fund these efforts.[x] Once a recruitment plan is developed for a specific study, the site should negotiate the budget for that plan separately. This helps the site direct the needed dollars specifically toward recruitment instead of derailing them into the general pot for other study activities. A separate budget also facilitates the tracking of the plan's success.

With or without a separate budget, some sites may be giving recruitment efforts short shrift. Results of a 1999 CenterWatch survey of 103 investigative sites revealed that sites spend only 7% of net revenue on patient recruitment initiatives.[xi] Some in the industry indicate that successful sites are more likely to be allocating as much as 15% to 17% of net revenue on patient recruitment.

The Nuts and Bolts of a Multi-Dimensional Patient Recruitment Campaign

Successful recruiting does not happen by accident. It requires extensive planning with the sponsor prior to study initiation, proper budgeting and a recognition that multi-dimensional recruitment techniques are often needed for each study (Table 1). As sophisticated sites embrace this philosophy, sites continuing with hackneyed one-size-fits-all methods are destined to be left behind. For example, relying solely on the in-house patient database may be sufficient for the site doing an occasional study, but sites aiming to expand operations need to consider broadening their approach.

When starting to structure the recruitment campaign, the target audience must be defined. Several key questions will help the recruitment team define the audience and select the modalities to support the campaign.[xii] These include:

- How many randomized patients are needed?
- For this therapeutic area, how many patients generally have to be screened to enroll the target number? (screen failure rate)
- What is the anticipated patient dropout rate?
- Does the sponsor and/or site have recent recruitment experience in this therapeutic category?
- What is the time frame from beginning to completion of enrollment?
- What is the incidence of this disease or condition?
- How onerous are the inclusion/exclusion criteria?
- What is the length of the study (i.e., treatment period)?
- How many sites are planned?
- What system is in place to handle the phone inquiries generated from the media campaign?
- Are competitive treatments already marketed?

Various Modalities Used to Recruit Patients
In-house patient database
Physician referral
Local newspaper
Radio
Television
Direct mail
Newsletter
Magazine
Internet
Centralized call centers
Speaking to community groups

Table 1

Answers to these questions will point the site toward certain campaign tactics. Studies for smoking cessation and for common conditions such as obesity, allergies during allergy season, soft tissue infection, acute back pain and osteoarthritis are relatively easy to fill and may signal using a combination of in-house database plus newspaper advertising to reach enrollment targets. Studies that often have more difficult inclusion/exclusion criteria, such as osteoporosis, heart failure, herpes zoster, stroke, outpatient pneumonia, rheumatoid arthritis and Alzheimer's disease, might warrant use of the in-house database, patient referral, newspaper, television and magazines. Whatever media mix is selected, the approach must be specific for each study, or at least for each therapeutic area. A campaign seeking post-menopausal women for a hormone replacement study would require a different strategy than the adolescent acne trial.

Recruitment advertisements are to be simple, direct and non-coercive. It is acceptable to state the disease or condition being studied; age range of the study subjects; benefits to the subject, namely the fact that the study item, study visits and all related tests and examinations are offered to subjects at no cost; and compensation, if any, for time and travel. Ads should also avoid any type of complex medical terminology (see ad on page 143).

For best results in broadcast ads, a female announcer should be used for studies requiring female subjects and a male announcer for studies requiring male subjects. Also, if you want to target a particular population that you know has a high incidence of the disease you're conducting a trial on, it is effective to have ads in the language of that population. For example, the Hispanic population has a high incidence of diabetes, and the Creole population has a high incidence of high cholesterol, so having radio ads for these types of trials in the respective languages of those populations and preferably on a radio program that has high demographics for those populations makes sense. Since African-Americans have a high incidence of hypertension, it's most effective to have an ad on a radio program that appeals to this audience.

Do you have

Low Back Pain?

You may be eligible to participate in a research study

18–75 years of age
Compensation for time and travel

Hip or Knee Pain?

Research Study

18 years of age or older
Have stiffness or pain
Compensation for time and travel

Migraine

Research Study

18–65 years of age
Comparing two over-the-counter pain relievers in investigational combinations
Compensation for time and travel

Psoriasis

Research Study

Documented history of psoriasis
Otherwise in good health
Compensation for time and travel

Qualified Program Participants Receive Study Related Care and Study Medication

Research Center

If prospective subjects are to be compensated for time and travel, this information may appear in the advertisement, but in small, non-bolded letters, preferably at the end of the ad. Large dollar signs or promises of earning "big bucks" for study participation are not acceptable.* Other guidelines for acceptable recruitment advertisements appear in Table 2.

Guidelines for Drafting Acceptable Patient Recruitment Advertisements
Advertise for "participants," "volunteers" or "study subjects," not for patients.
Avoid phrases such as "receive new treatment," "new medication" or "new drug" as they suggest that the study item is a newly marketed product with proven worth. It is better to use "investigational" or "research."
Advertisements should not promise "free medical treatment," when the intent is only to say subjects will not be charged for participating in the investigation.
It is acceptable to include the name, address and phone number of the clinical investigator and/or research facility, as well as the name of person or office to contact for further information.
Advertising for study volunteers is a reflection of the informed consent form. Information not contained in the informed consent forms is not to be included.
Ads may state that the subject will be compensated for time and travel, but should not emphasize the compensatory benefits of participation. The amount of compensation to participants should not be coercive or present undue influence. Statement of payment should be the last information given. It should not be enlarged or bolded or include large dollar signs.
Submit advertisements that are being taped for broadcase to the IRB for review before the final audio/videotape is produced. The IRB may review and approve the wording of the ad before taping, which precludes having to re-tape due to inappropriate content.

Table 2 Source: Guidance for IRBs and Clinical Investigators, Palm Beach Research Center

* Payment to research subjects for participation in studies is not considered a benefit, but a recruitment incentive. The amount and schedule of all payments should be presented to the IRB at the time of initial review. The IRB will review both to assure that neither is coercive or presents undue influence (21CFR Part 50.20).

A Word About Informed Consent

The FDA considers advertising for study subjects as the start of the Informed Consent process. This is reflected in the agency's expectation that IRBs will review all research documents and activities that bear directly on the rights and welfare of the proposed subjects.
Informed Consent is a fundamental mechanism to ensure respect for persons through provision of thoughtful consent for a voluntary act. The language of informed consent, especially explanation of the study's procedures, alternatives, risks and benefits is to be written in lay language. Obtaining informed consent is the responsibility of the investigator (21 Code of Federal Regulations–CFR Part 312.60).
Basic elements of Informed Consent (21 CFR Part 50.25) include: A statement that the study involves research
An explanation of the purposes of the research
The expected duration of the subject's participation
A description of the procedures to be followed
Identification of any procedures that are experimental
A description of any reasonably foreseeable risks or discomforts to the subject
A description of any benefits to the subjects or to others which may reasonably be expected from the research
A disclosure of appropriate alternative procedures or courses of treatment, if any, that might be advantageous to the subject
A statement describing the extent, if any, to which confidentiality of records identifying the subject be maintained
For research involving more than minimal risk, an explanation as to whether any compensation, and an explanation as to whether any medical treatments are available, if injury occurs and, if so, what they consist of, or where further information may be obtained
An explanation of whom to contact for answers to pertinent questions about the research and research subjects' rights, and whom to contact in the event of a research-related injury
A statement that participation is voluntary, refusal to participate will involve no penalty or loss of benefits to which the subject is otherwise entitled, and the subject may discontinue participation at any time without penalty or loss of benefits, to which the subject is otherwise entitled.

Source: Office of Human Research Protection
http://ohrp.osophs.dhhs.gov/humansubjects/assurance/consentckls.htm

Before they appear in print or on the airwaves, all recruitment advertisements to be seen or heard by prospective subjects to solicit their participation are to be submitted to the study's institutional review board (IRB). Because the Food and Drug Administration (FDA) considers direct advertising for study subjects to be the start of the informed consent and subject selection processes, advertisements should be reviewed and approved by the IRB as part of the package for initial review.[xiii] The IRB, charged with ensuring that appropriate safeguards exist to protect the rights and welfare of research subjects,** will determine if the ads are coercive or if they imply a certainty of favorable outcome beyond what is outlined in the informed consent document and in the protocol.

At Palm Beach Research Center, we have learned through extensive trial and error which tactics work for which type of study. Newspaper advertising seems to be most effective for studies for which the patient can self-diagnose, such as obesity, back pain or migraine headache, or for a condition the patient knows he or she has, such as osteoarthritis, psoriasis or diabetes. When we opt for newspaper advertising, we place the ads in the front section, preferably on page 2. We've been successful using the local edition of *Shopper's Guide*, placing the announcements on the inside back cover, sometimes describing several studies in the same ad. *Shopper's Guide* is not a national publication, but many cities and towns have something comparable to it that can be inserted into a newspaper, such as a *Pennysaver* or a little coupon newspaper that is distributed door-to-door. Most people read it looking for sales and bargains. Ads outlined in purple seem to attract attention. When recruiting for women's studies, we've found that a graphic of a rose is an attention getter. For arthritis studies, displaying a picture of a knee grabs the reader's interest.

Recruiting Situations that Respond Well to Advertising
Very common disease state
Patient can self-diagnose
Patient knows he or she has a specific condition
Patient is self-treating
Patient's current medication is not fully satisfactory
Patient has difficulty receiving adequate treatment for condition

Table 3

** 21 Code of Federal Regulations (CFR) 56.107(a) and 21 CFR 56.111.

Television can be very powerful and successful. For the appropriate studies, it can be more effective than print media, dollar for dollar, in terms of yielding enrolled subjects.[xiv] Other recruiting situations that respond well to advertising are listed in Table 3. TV ads should be used for studies of the most common diseases. For example, osteoarthritis has a much larger patient population than rheumatoid arthritis. This population is usually elderly and a mix of men and women, so we look at the demographics of different TV shows and advertise on shows with a demographic that matches the demographics of the population we need to recruit.

We have experienced uneven results with radio advertising. This method can only be useful when advertising at a time when prospective candidates are likely to be home and can scribble the phone number when it is mentioned.

Additional strategies we use include:

- In-house database of research patients
- Quarterly newsletter to research database
- Periodic faxes to area physicians announcing ongoing and upcoming trials
- Cross-study recruitment
- Making our private practice patients aware of studies through bulletin board postings and flyers
- Giving talks that carry continuing medical education (CME) units for physicians (Sometimes, the sponsor provides slides.)
- Educating area pharmacists of ongoing studies, and leaving flyers at the counters (National headquarters of the large chains often must be contacted first.)
- Writing brief articles for organizations such as the American Heart Association, American Cancer Society, etc.
- Participating in local medical radio talk shows
- Contacting public health clinics and emergency rooms about studies.

A few of these techniques are discussed below in greater detail.

In-House Research Database

Investigators may have thousands of patient charts in their private practice, but those charts are likely to be in paper form. For this reason, they are not easily searchable for purposes of clinical trials, unless the physician is unusually familiar with his or her patients or staff is available to review the charts, looking for ICD-9 diagnoses that may identify patients likely to meet eligibility criteria. Also, private practice databases consist of patients who may have little or no interest in clinical trials and may not appreciate their private medical information being used for recruitment purposes. The patient database from your practice can be a good way to start recruiting patients, especially if you are a small site. The important thing is to show respect for patient confidentiality by having the physician contact the patient first to determine whether the patient is open to the idea of participating in a study.

Another way to approach patients in your database is to mail post cards to all of them asking them if they would be interested in participating in clinical trials or being notified of future trials. The post card can have a checklist of conditions that they have or trials they would be interested in so that when they send in their cards, you can place them on a separate research database. Then you can send them a newsletter or post cards when different studies become available so that they can be screened for them. Research databases consist of people who have responded to advertisements, community presentations or to their physicians' suggestion that they consider a specific study.

At PBRC, we maintain a separate research database. Information is entered into the database electronically by our phone screeners as they speak to prospective candidates calling in response to advertising. Data on patients who fail the phone screen are saved in the database.

PBRC further develops the research database by sponsoring booths at Senior Health Fairs or giving community presentations about clinical trials in specific therapeutic areas. At those events, attendees who express interest in clinical trials are asked to complete a Patient Data Form, with the understanding that the information will be added to a research database (See Appendix).

Because our database is searchable, it is an invaluable source of information to be mined for future studies. Once candidates with specific conditions are identified, recruitment post cards or letters can be sent, often yielding a good response. In addition, many sponsors are willing to cover the cost of database mailings, a factor the site should consider as it develops the costs of a patient recruitment campaign.

Database Newsletter

Newsletters educate patients about various disease and health conditions and disseminate information about currently enrolling studies. At PBRC, we send quarterly newsletters to our entire research database, an activity that has proven to be an effective recruiting tactic. All study-related information is approved by the sponsors and by the IRB. Invariably, the newsletter generates lots of telephone calls. It also serves to keep our database updated in two ways. First, a caller may notify us of a new address, a change that our phone screeners make immediately, and secondly, newsletters with old addresses are returned to us, sometimes with information about the new address.

Periodic Faxes to Area Physicians

Periodically, PBRC faxes a different sort of newsletter to area doctors' offices to inform them of ongoing and upcoming trials. The purpose of this newsletter is to seek referrals for the listed studies. Although physicians in the community are often reluctant to refer a patient, for fear of losing that patient and the associated revenue, some familiar with PBRC will refer if they recognize that a study offers their patients an opportunity to receive treatment for conditions for which there is no good presently marketed alternative. Our physician newsletter has resulted in numerous referrals and has led several physicians to visit our site to learn more about our operations. A few have ended up becoming our sub-investigators.

Cross-Study Recruitment

This approach enhances recruitment efforts by using several techniques. First, it involves informing current study participants of other studies that may be of interest, following the proper break period between two studies. This is a good approach because current subjects are familiar with the clinical trials process and may be inclined to consider further studies or spread the word to friends and family, especially if they enjoyed a positive experience with the first one.

Cross-study recruitment also encourages prospective subjects who are disqualified from one study to consider a different one. In order for this to be effective, recruiters must be aware of the other studies taking place, or else the computer system they are using must be able to default to another study for which the caller fits the entrance criteria.

At PBRC, we have found that the database newsletter used in concert with cross-study recruitment is a powerful recruiting tool. Oftentimes, someone responds to a study mentioned in the newsletter, and although he or she does not qualify for that study, that person may be screened for others for possible eligibility.

National Recruitment Campaigns

When orchestrating recruitment efforts, the site will need to consider whether the sponsor is designing a national media campaign for a study. If so, the site should designate someone to work with the sponsor to ensure placement of ads in the proper print media, and if broadcasts are used, on the most appropriate radio and television stations. In addition, the site needs to know if the sponsor is working with specific organizations, such as the American Diabetes Association or the American Heart Association. Information about the studies might appear on the web sites of those associations or in publications of interest to prospective subjects. When negotiating the budget for a new study, the site needs to ask the sponsor if it plans a national media campaign, and if so, what the nature of that campaign is expected to be. This can help the site develop its budget for recruitment activities.

Newer Methods of Recruiting

Tried and true methods of recruiting such as internal patient database, physician referral, print and broadcast media, and direct mail are still the mainstay of recruiting activities, but some less traditional tools are starting to emerge. The Internet, professional patient recruitment providers and centralized call centers are some of the up and coming strategies.

As recently as the early 1990s, virtually no companies were offering Internet-based patient recruitment solutions. By the mid-1990s, the landscape starting changing as some patient recruitment contractors began including the Web among a variety of media used to reach potential patients.[xv] At that time, the Web was used mostly to post summaries of ongoing trials and contact information. More recently, interactive web sites have become widespread, allowing interested parties to submit their names, demographic data and possibly some pre-screening information online. Prospective patients can also send emails to the web site to request additional information.

As long as the web site limits information to providing the title of the study, purpose of the study, protocol summary, basic eligibility criteria, study site location and how to contact the site, IRB review and approval are not required.[xvi] If, however, other descriptive information is added, IRB review and approval are needed to assure that the additional information does not promise or imply a certainty of cure or other benefit beyond what is contained in the protocol and the informed consent document.

The array of web sites offering clinical trials information continues to change, but as of this writing, some of the players are:***

- *www.acurian.com*
- *www.cancernet.nci.nih.gov*
- *www.centerwatch.com*
- *www.clinicaltrials.com*
- *www.clinicaltrials.gov*
- *www.ecancertrials.com*
- *www.emergingmed.com* (cancer trials)
- *www.hopelink.com*
- *www.veritasmedicine.com*

In addition to these Internet trial listing services, some sites, site management organizations and sponsors post their ongoing and upcoming trials on their own interactive web sites.

While it is not clear how effective the Internet is at turning web surfers into enrollees, there is anecdotal evidence suggesting that it is playing a growing role. A study of 1050 study volunteers showed that 9% of them learned of their study on the Internet.[xvii] In another case, a major pharmaceutical firm used a multi-media approach, including the Internet, to disseminate information about a pivotal forty-center trial for an antidepressant. At the conclusion of the study, the sponsor determined that 16% of the 1000 randomized patients who completed the trial resulted from that

*** As of August 2001, some of these web sites are interactive while others post information about the studies and contact information.

Internet listing. The sponsor also calculated that it had spent approximately $63 per enrolled patient through the Internet—less than half the per-patient spending for several other recruitment approaches implemented.[xviii]

The Internet has spawned a new group of clinical service providers that charge sponsors a fee to match visitors of specific clinical trials web sites to sponsors of those trials.[xix] The services work by having prospective trial volunteers complete online questionnaires that contain eligibility criteria for specific trials. If a completed questionnaire seems to match the most basic eligibility criteria, the Internet "matchmaker" forwards the information to the trial's sponsor. Once the sponsor determines that the candidate should be considered for pre-screening, the matchmaker company will provide the patient with contact information to reach either an investigative site or a centralized call center. The service is free to prospective patients.

To drive potential candidates to sites posting trials, the matchmakers develop or license content on numerous therapeutic areas. They may also offer chat groups, place hyperlinks on other sites with an established high traffic base, or offer other interactive services.

These Internet matchmakers are the latest version of patient recruitment companies, organizations that specialize in developing multi-media campaigns to meet enrollment targets, usually for multi-center trials. Prior to structuring an advertising campaign, these vendors attempt to uncover the motivations of potential subjects, and then work with the clients to attract those subjects by addressing their wants and needs. Because of their expertise in this area, professional recruiters are knowledgeable about the costs associated with drafting appropriate campaigns. If they have experience in the therapeutic area of interest, they may also be able to project the number of inquiries needed to result in one enrolled patient.

Professional recruitment companies may be hired by sponsors, or if enrollment responsibilities have been delegated, by the contracted CROs or, on rare occasions, site management organizations (SMOs). These recruiters also offer implementation services and programs to retain enrolled subjects. Generally, the individual site does not employ patient recruitment companies as they tend to focus on large, national campaigns. The free-standing site may, however, be the beneficiary of one of these national campaigns if the site is participating in the study of interest.

Recruitment vendors commonly use centralized call centers as part of a multi-center recruitment strategy. As in many industries, call centers play an important role in fielding thousands of calls, an activity that is beyond the capability of the average business. In the clinical trials industry, the typical site can be too overwhelmed by the dozens of screening calls that come in from advertisements. Each call is important, and each person deserves to have his or her questions answered, yet busy sites are often ill-prepared to perform this function. In addition, if a caller leaves a message at the site and that call is not returned, or returned days later, the subject is likely to be disillusioned with the process.

Patient recruitment call centers are designed to handle several key functions such as:

- Pre-screening prospective subjects who are responding to advertisements through the use of standardized scripts
- Forwarding names to investigative sites of prospective candidates who passed the telephone screen
- Scheduling and reminding patients of study appointments
- Calling patients to encourage study compliance
- Gathering patient feedback during and after the trial
- Providing management reports on total number of responses to media, the ratio of preliminary phone screen passes to fails, the success of various media, etc.

As call center functions become more integrated with Internet operations, they will be able to manage the entire online communication process, linking study subjects to the sites. For example, the call center will be able to provide content online to the prospective candidate, along with useful web addresses, answers to questions through web chat, and emails on trials in therapeutic areas of interest.

CenterWatch estimates that sponsors are spending approximately $50 million to $55 million annually on the thirty-some call centers with patient recruitment capability.[xx] In addition, some of the large sites, and some SMOs have established in-house call center functions. PBRC set up a four-person call center a few years ago and believes the operation speeds the screening process and enables the company to offer a high level of customer service. Creating a positive first impression of the site is the first step in the recruitment process.

Metrics

Once a recruitment campaign begins, it is important to measure its ongoing success. Constantly evaluating the campaign as it unfolds helps to identify the more productive efforts and redirect less effective ones. At the conclusion of the campaign, data should be tallied to determine overall campaign success by media type, the number of candidates that had to be screened to yield one enrolled, randomized patient, and the cost of randomization by media type (Table 4).

Metrics are important not only to identify winning patient recruitment strategies but also to help sites substantiate their claims to sponsors that they are able to meet enrollment targets in accordance with the negotiated timeframe. In a marketplace where competition for studies is very keen, sponsors need ways to distinguish among sites vying for the same studies. Sites with

Advertising Effectiveness for One Site

Media Source	Description	Study	Calls	Prescreen	Screen	Randomized	% Randomized	Event Cost	Cost Per Call	Cost Per Randomization
950 KJR AM	Evening Spot	93213	14	7	7	5	35.71%	$5,000	$357	$1,000
Telethon Services	Telephone Campaign	93213	16	10	10	9	56.25%	$8,500	$531	$944.44
Fox Q13	Lunchtime Ad	2342	19	6	6	3	15.79%	$7,500	$394	$2,500
Seattle Times	1 month half-page ad	954-410	12	6	6	4	33.33%	$2,000	$167	$500
Washington Asthma Alliance	Speaking Engagement Monthly Mtg.	954-410	10	6	6	2	20.00%	$1,150	$115	$575
www.nwresearch.com	Web Site	A-9192	24	10	10	8	33.33%	$5,000	$208	$625
Site Totals			**95**	**45**	**45**	**31**		**$29,150**		

Table 4 Source: Advanced Clinical Software

documented track records may stand out over those claiming ability to enroll but cannot produce any documentation beyond verbal assurance.

Metrics are not infallible, however. They show successes of past studies with entrance criteria that are invariably different from those of new studies. Eligibility criteria for new studies may be easier or more difficult than those previously conducted by the site. For this reason, metrics are not a predictor of future success. They are perhaps most useful when grouped by therapeutic areas. Metrics documenting Site A's ten successful phase III migraine headache studies may be a better indicator than Site B's combined metrics of thirty unrelated studies in projecting a site's future effectiveness with a new phase III migraine study. Although metrics cannot predict future achievement, Site A may have the better chance of procuring that new migraine study.

Sites can easily start keeping metrics by using ordinary word processing or accounting packages. Commercially available recruiting software is also available. These products generally offer coordinated modules for recruitment, budgeting, database management, appointment scheduling and reminder letters. At this time, the keeping of metrics is not a widespread practice and, at some sites, may consist of little more than data collected from one successful study, or the number of calls resulting from advertising. There is neither a body of literature nor industry standards to benchmark metrics.[xxi] In the interim, sites that attempt to document their successes, particularly in specific therapeutic areas, may enhance their abilities to attract new studies.

The Clinical Trial Volunteer

The patient recruitment process is designed to attract, enroll, randomize and retain the clinical trial volunteer. A whole industry is growing up around these efforts. Patient recruitment companies, Internet recruitment vendors, centralized call centers, protocol feasibility vendors and in-house marketing staff are working with sponsors, CROs, SMOs and independent sites to find and keep that elusive patient.

Difficulty in finding patients stems not only from the burgeoning number of trials seeking volunteers but also from the mass media, which have reported many negative news stories about clinical trials. Prospective study subjects are not likely to volunteer if they hold a negative impression of any aspect of the industry. They need to perceive the clinical trials industry as safe, ethical and trustworthy.

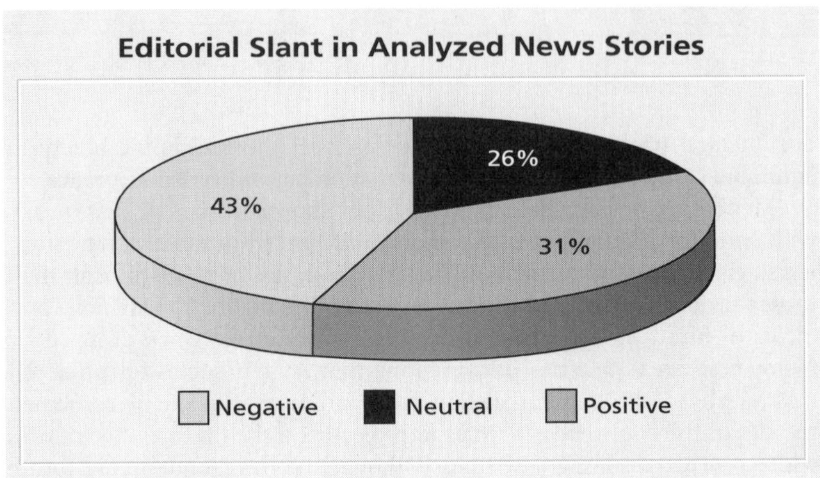

Figure 2 Source: Association of Clinical Research Professionals (ACRP)

The Association of Clinical Research Professionals (ACRP) Future Trends Committee conducted two non-scientific studies, looking at the slant of news stories about clinical research.[xxii] The first study evaluated 100 articles that appeared in 1999 or 2000 in major publications such as *The New York Times*, *The Los Angeles Times*, *The Washington Post*, *The Seattle Times* and *USA Today*. The articles were rated as either positive, negative or neutral (Figure 2).

Positive articles tended to focus mostly on gains made in fighting particular diseases, and had titles such as:

- "Alzheimer's vaccine study promising"[xxiii]
- "Treatment for cancer advances in trials"[xxiv]
- "A promising weapon in the fight against MS"[xxv]

Neutral articles dealt with business news pertaining to sponsors, information about the clinical trials process or government regulation of drug studies. Negative stories addressed a wide array of issues and outnumbered the other two categories. Some of these titles included:

- "A doctor's drug trials turn into fraud"[xxvi]
- "Cheaters may seriously skew clinical trial results"[xxvii]
- "How a new policy led to seven deadly drugs"[xxviii]
- "The biotech death of Jesse Gelsinger"[xxix]

The second analysis looked at 75 articles published between January 2000 and January 2001 in *The Los Angeles Times*, *The Washington Post*, *The Chicago Tribune*, *The Dallas Morning News*, *The Philadelphia Inquirer* and *USA Today*. This review did not include articles about business aspects of clinical trials or recent advances in specific therapeutic areas. It did focus on articles discussing regulatory enforcement, patient safety and investigator conflicts of interest. The articles were assessed as to whether they would encourage or discourage the reader from volunteering for a trial. In this study, 55 of the 75 articles, 74%, were deemed as having a negative impact.

In stark contrast to the negative press, participants in clinical trials report having very positive experiences. CenterWatch conducted two separate studies on the subject of patient satisfaction. The first one, in 1999, surveyed 210 subjects and found a high level of satisfaction with their study participation (Figure 3).[xxx] Eighty-seven percent (87%) rated their overall care as either "excellent" or "good." Ninety-one percent (91%) reported that their care was as good or better than that which they received from their primary care physician. Importantly, 77% said they would "definitely" participate in a clinical trial again.

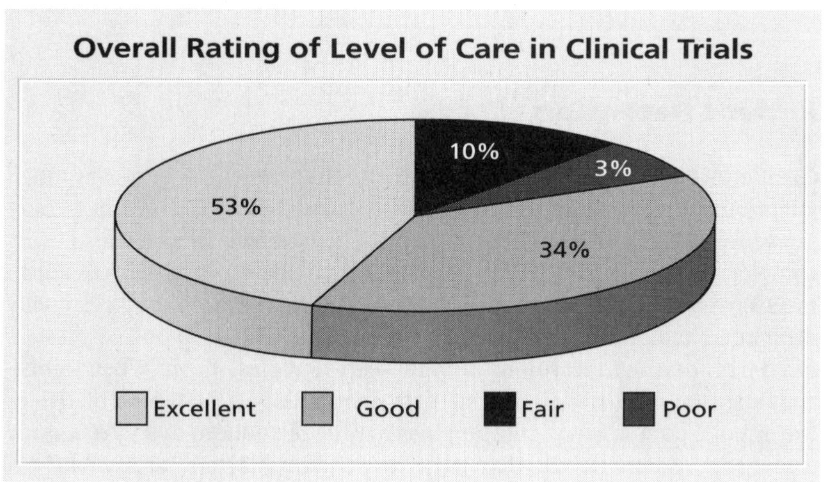

Figure 3 Source: CenterWatch 1999

The second study on patient satisfaction was conducted between April 1999 and March 2000, and included 1050 randomly selected participants. It revealed similar positive experiences. In this study, 90% rated their overall quality of care as either "excellent" or "good" (Figure 4), and 75% stated they would "definitely" participate in another clinical trial. Respondents also provided feedback as to areas of their clinical experience that needed improvement. Thirty-one percent cited better de-briefing and post-study follow-up as the areas most in need of improvement.

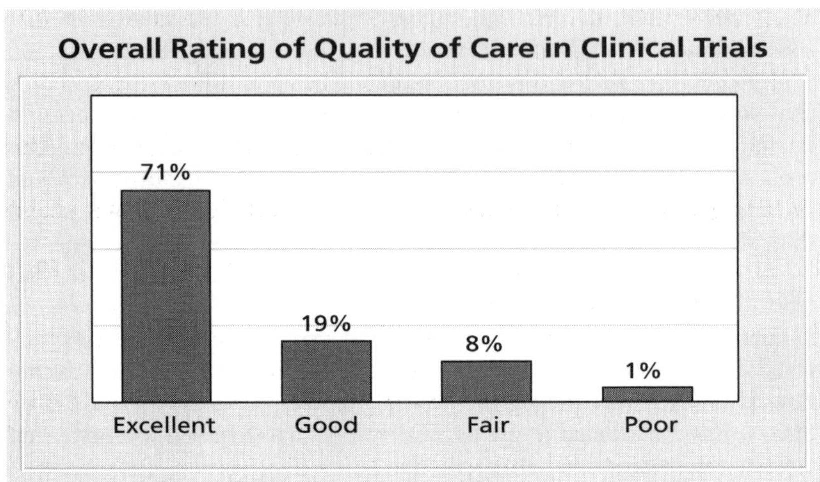

Figure 4 Source: CenterWatch 2000

Patient Retention

Great effort is expended recruiting and enrolling patients, but just as much attention should be paid to patient retention. On average, only one person in twenty who responds to a recruitment solicitation or referral will actually complete a clinical trial.[****,xxxi] While some of these prospects will fail to meet eligibility criteria, others will enroll, be randomized, but eventually drop out. Data cannot be collected from patients who drop out, so sites are faced with having to recruit more volunteers to replace them. When significant attrition occurs, the resulting data may no longer be representative of the original population, significant bias may be introduced that affects study finding and generalizability to a larger population may not be possible.[xxxii]

Patient retention is a natural by-product of patient satisfaction. The satisfaction process starts with treating patients with respect and honesty from the very first contact and extending throughout the trial.[xxxiii] Each contact

**** This is an average. Rates vary by disease.

that the subject has with the site contributes to the possibility of continued participation or withdrawal. Consequently, everyone at the staff needs to make the patient feel special at each study visit. This means being friendly, professional and knowledgeable. It means doing more than merely going through the mechanics required of each study visit. The site can take extra steps such as keeping patients informed about the trial's progress and offering information about their conditions. Volunteers may find this empowering, a positive feeling that could affect their decision to remain in the trial. Additionally, subjects who complete the trial, having had a good experience along the way, are often receptive to participating in future studies and may spread the word to friends and family.

Some patients have logistical problems that could hinder their ability to keep study appointments. Sites may consider offering onsite day care if they foresee conducting a large number of studies targeting young women. This service may be critical for the retention of some mothers of young children. Providing round trip transportation for older participants might enable them to remain in the study.

Other important tactics that can boost retention include mailing reminder cards for upcoming visits or simply calling the day before the scheduled appointment. Increasingly, email may be used for this function. Following a study, the site may want to mail an evaluation form to each candidate to solicit opinion of his or her experience. Information gleaned from these forms can be used to improve the quality of the patient's experience.

The receptionist answering the telephone should know which trials are being conducted and the names of the coordinators for each study. It is a good idea to keep a list of the current studies near the telephones. Without this mechanism, patients and prospective patients calling the site may be greeted by a receptionist who is unaware of the ongoing studies. This can be discouraging to callers, especially those who were nervous about placing that initial call. It also sounds unprofessional and sends a signal that the site is disorganized.

In Review

Patient recruitment and enrollment remain among the most challenging activities for sites as the number of studies in the United States rises to 50,000 to 60,000 annually and the number of patients per new drug application approaches 4,400. Meeting this challenge calls for the use of multidimensional, targeted recruitment strategies. Relying on a few limited approaches for all studies, such as the in-house patient database and the occasional newspaper advertisement and radio campaign, is often insufficient in today's competitive market. A more professional, broad-based effort needs to be expended prior to study initiation.

When starting patient recruitment planning, the first step is to define the target audience. This can be accomplished by answering a series of questions designed to determine the media venues best suited to enroll the study at hand. How many randomized patients are needed? For this therapeutic area, how many patients generally have to be screened to enroll the target number? What is the anticipated patient dropout rate? How onerous are the inclusion/exclusion criteria?

Answers to these questions and others point to certain campaign designs specific for each study. They may include various mixes of in-house patient database, newspaper, television, Internet, direct mail and health fairs. Once the campaign is mapped out and costed out, budgeting for this effort should be negotiated separately from the main study budget. Creating a separate budget for study recruitment underscores the importance of this activity and reduces the possibility that recruitment funds will be re-directed to other study-related efforts.

Developing community awareness of your site can facilitate recruitment success. Sending periodic newsletters to the research database and to local physicians about ongoing and upcoming studies will increase name recognition and familiarize the community with the type of work that takes place at your site. Speaking to groups of physicians about specific therapeutic areas or speaking to community groups about clinical research will achieve the same result. The hope is that the name familiarity will eventually lead some consumers to call for pre-screening and some physicians to refer potential subjects. A few physicians may even express interest in becoming sub-investigators. This community effort may also serve to counteract some of the negative image of clinical research perpetrated by the mass media. Indeed, research suggests that most study participants have an overwhelmingly positive experience and three-quarters would definitely participate in another study.

Retention of volunteers goes hand-in-hand with recruitment and enrollment efforts. As the recruitment campaign unfolds, all prospective subjects are to be treated with respect and dignity every step of the way. Treating them in this fashion and providing the best quality of care during the screening, enrollment and randomization phases can go a long way toward retaining patients.

And finally, a site that invests in the expense of a well-designed recruitment campaign needs to account for the campaign's success through the keeping of metrics. Over time, keeping metrics builds a history for the site that it can share with sponsors seeking to place studies at sites with a proven record of reaching enrollment targets in accordance with a negotiated timeline. Because the keeping of metrics is still relatively new, sites that keep them to document success may be better positioned to attract studies than those that lack comparable records.

The issue of patient recruitment is a complex one. Prospective subjects must be attracted to the study, qualify, enroll, be randomized and be retained. While all of this requires a great deal of dedication, strategizing and organization by the site, the effort can be facilitated by the realization that many volunteers feel a certain reward in being able to help others. People volunteer primarily to seek help for conditions that are not treated satisfactorily with currently marketed products. Many also want to help advance science.

References

[i] *A Guide to Patient Recruitment, Today's Best Practices and Strategies,* Diana Anderson, Ph.D., CenterWatch, Inc., 2001, p. 11.

[ii] CenterWatch, Boston, Mass., May 2000.

[iii] Tufts Center for the Study of Drug Development, 1999; *Food and Drug Law Journal,* C. Peck, 1997.

[iv] "Grant Market to Exceed $4 Billion in 2000," *CenterWatch,* November 2000, Vol. 7, Issue 11, p. 9.

[v] Ibid., *CenterWatch,* p. 9.

[vi] Barnett International, 2000.

[vii] "Series of reports prompted reforms in human research," Edward T. Pound, *USA Today,* June 12, 2000, p. 9A.

[viii] "Surfing for Study Subjects," *CenterWatch,* February 2000, Vol. 7, Issue 2, Lisa Henderson, p. 6.

[ix] "A Look at the Internet's Patient Recruitment Matchmakers," *CenterWatch,* Vol. 8, Issue 7, Whitney Allen, p. 8.

[x] *A Guide to Patient Recruitment, Today's Best Practices and Strategies,* Diana Anderson, Ph.D., CenterWatch, Inc., 2001, pp. 13-14.

[xi] "Sites Prosper...but Financial Health Threatened," *CenterWatch,* Vol. 7, Issue 1, January 2000, p. 11.

[xii] *A Guide to Patient Recruitment, Today's Best Practices and Strategies,* Diana Anderson, Ph.D., CenterWatch, Inc., 2001, pp. 75-76, 145-146.

[xiii] *Guidance for IRBs and Clinical Investigators, www.fda.gov/oc/ohrt/irbs/toc4.html#recruiting,* accessed August 24, 2001.

[xiv] Healthcare Communications Group, 2001.

[xv] "Surfing for Study Subjects," *CenterWatch,* February 2000, Vol. 7, Issue 2, Lisa Henderson, pp. 5-6.

[xvi] *Guidance for IRBs and Clinical Investigators, www.fda.gov/oc/ohrt/irbs/toc4.html#recruiting,* accessed August 24, 2001.

[xvii] CenterWatch's 2000 survey of 1050 study volunteers.

[xviii] *A Guide to Patient Recruitment, Today's Best Practices and Strategies,* Diana Anderson, Ph.D., CenterWatch, Inc., 2001, p. 178.

[xix] "A Look at the Internet's Patient Recruitment Matchmakers," *CenterWatch,* Vol. 8, Issue 7, Whitney Allen, p. 9.

[xx] "Call Centers Dial Up For Patients," *CenterWatch,* March 2001, Vol. 8, Issue 3, Steve Zisson, p. 6.

[xxi] *A Guide to Patient Recruitment, Today's Best Practices and Strategies,* Diana Anderson, Ph.D., CenterWatch, Inc., 2001, p. 98.

[xxii] "Clinical Research in Transition," *The Monitor*, Association of Clinical Research Professionals (ACRP), Summer 2001, Vol. 15, Issue 2, James W. Maloy et al., pp. 35, 36.

[xxiii] "Alzheimer's vaccine study promising,"Sally Squires, *The Washington Post*, Section A, July 12, 2000.

[xxiv] "Treatment for cancer advances in trials," Nicholas Wade, *The New York Times*, Health & Fitness, August 1, 2000.

[xxv] "A promising weapon in the fight against MS," Judy Silber, *The Los Angeles Times*, Metro, September 7, 2000.

[xxvi] "A doctor's drug trials turn into fraud," Kurt Eichenwald and Gina Kolata, *The New York Times*, Business/Financial, May 17, 1999.

[xxvii] "Cheaters may seriously skew clinical trial results", Thomas Maugh II, *The Los Angeles Times*, Health Section, August 21, 2000.

[xxviii] "How a new policy led to seven deadly drugs," David Willman, *The Los Angeles Times*, Section A, December 9, 1999.

[xxix] "The biotech death of Jesse Gelsinger," Sheryl Gay Stolberg, *The New York Times Magazine*, November 28, 1999.

[xxx] "A Word From Clinical Trial Volunteers," *CenterWatch*, June 1999, Vol. 6, Issue 6, pp. 1, 9-13.

[xxxi] "Grant Market to Exceed $4 Billion in 2000," *CenterWatch*, November 2000, Vol. 7, Issue 11, p. 9.

[xxxii] "Subject Loss in Infancy Research: How Biasing is it?" *Infant Behavior and Development*, G.A. Richardson & K.A. McCluskey, 1983, pp. 235-239.

[xxxiii] *A Guide to Patient Recruitment, Today's Best Practices and Strategies,* Diana Anderson, Ph.D., CenterWatch, Inc., 2001, p. 213.

CHAPTER 11

Patient Protection

- An Overview of Ethical Guidelines
- Ethical Guidelines at the Site Level
- Federal Oversight
- In Review

Investigators who commit ethical violations are unwittingly violating essential protections needed to keep volunteers safe. For this reason, the training of new investigators and ongoing training for experienced investigators should include a background in ethics. Without education in this subject, investigators may lack an understanding of the importance of regulations designed to safeguard patients and prevent coercive practice. Investigators may also be unaware of the history behind their derivation.

An Overview of Ethical Guidelines

In the United States, the field of ethics in clinical research has its basis in both international and national guidelines. Extending back more than fifty years, they reflect efforts to standardize international clinical research practices involving human volunteers. They include:

- The Nuremberg Code
- The Declaration of Helsinki

- The Belmont Report
- The International Conference on Harmonization (ICH)

On the international level, the Nuremberg Code and the Declaration of Helsinki form the backbone of contemporary ethical standards, addressing issues of informed consent and human subject protections. The Nuremberg Code of 1947 was part of the judgment handed down by the war tribunal following Nazi atrocities committed in World War II, including cruel human experimentation.[i] The Code contains ten principles to which physicians must conform when performing experiments on human subjects. The first principle establishes that informed consent must be given freely by prospective subjects, without coercion (Table 1). Other principles in the Code describe how to take precautions to prevent unnecessary mental and physical suffering by subjects, and that research should be conducted by scientifically qualified staff.

First Principle of the Nuremberg Code

The voluntary consent of the human subject is absolutely essential. This means that the person involved should have legal capacity to give consent, should be so situated as to be able to exercise free power of choice, without the intervention of any element of force, fraud, deceit, duress, overreaching, or ulterior form of constraint or coercion; and should have sufficient knowledge and comprehension of the elements of the subject matter involved as to enable him to make an understanding and enlightened decision. This latter element requires that before the acceptance of an affirmative decision by the experimental subject there should be made known to him the nature and duration and purpose of the experiment; the method and means by which it is to be conducted; all inconveniences and hazards reasonably to be expected; and the effects upon his health or person which may possibly come from his participation in the experiment.

The duty and responsibility for ascertaining the quality of the consent rests upon each individual who initiates, directs or engages in the experiment. It is a personal duty and responsibility which may not be delegated to another with impunity.

Table 1 Source: Nuremberg Code

The Declaration of Helsinki was first adopted in 1964 by the World Medical Association (WMA) and has been revised several times,[ii] most recently in October 2000. Since 1964, the Declaration has evolved from a relatively broad set of ethical principles into a more defined, prescriptive set of guidelines addressing numerous subject protections and investigator responsibilities. Several of the guidelines appear in Table 2.

Several Guidelines of the Declaration of Helsinki
In medical research on human subjects, considerations related to the well-being of the human subject should take precedence over the interests of science and society.
Medical research is subject to ethical standards that promote respect for all human beings and protect their health and rights. Some research populations are vulnerable and need special protection. The particular needs of the economically and medically disadvantaged must be recognized.
Every medical research project involving human subjects should be preceded by careful assessment of predictable risks and burdens and comparison with foreseeable benefits to the subject or to others. This does not preclude the participation of healthy volunteers in medical research. The design of all studies should be publicly available.

Table 2 Source: World Medical Assembly, October 2000

In 1974, the National Research Act (Public Law 93-348) was signed into law, thereby creating the National Commission for the Protection of Human Subjects of Biomedical and Behavioral Research. The Commission drafted *Ethical Principles and Guidelines for the Protection of Human Subjects of Research*, commonly known as the Belmont Report.[iii] This report, which was published in the Federal Register in 1979, contains the three basic ethical principles upon which the federal regulations for protection of human subjects are based. They are:

- Respect for Persons
- Beneficence
- Justice

Respect for Persons incorporates two ethical convictions: first, that individuals should be treated as autonomous agents capable of deliberating about personal goals; and second, that persons with diminished autonomy are entitled to increased protections. This latter group refers to vulnerable populations who cannot participate fully in the informed consent process, such as children, some mentally disabled, individuals with dementia and other cognitive disorders and prisoners.

In the Belmont report, Beneficence refers to acts of kindness or charity that are the obligation of clinical professionals. They are to treat volunteers in an ethical manner not only by respecting their decisions and protecting them from harm, but also by making efforts to secure their well-being. Two general rules have been formulated as expressions of beneficent actions: do no harm; and maximize possible benefits while minimizing possible harms. This last action forms the basis for the regulatory requirement to perform risk/benefit assessments.

The principle of Justice asks the question, "Who ought to receive the benefits of research and who ought to bear its burdens?" This principle looks at the sense of fairness in distribution of benefits. Justice demands that research should not unduly involve people from groups unlikely to be among the beneficiaries of subsequent applications of the research. For example, in the past, the burdens of serving as research subjects fell largely upon the poor, while the benefits of improved medical care flowed primarily to private patients. In addition, the selection of research subjects should not systematically draw from certain classes, such as particular ethnic minorities or persons confined to institutions, simply because they are more easily available than others. Finally, this principle requires inclusion of diverse populations so that they may participate equally and benefit from the findings of research.

Many of these principles, which flow directly from the Nuremberg Code, are included in a succession of policies known as the Common Rule. They reflect current U.S. policy for protection of human research subjects as detailed in 45 Code of Federal Regulations Part 46 Subpart A. The Common Rule has been promulgated by seventeen different federal departments and independent agencies.

The International Conference on Harmonization (ICH), initiated in 1990, is a joint initiative between regulators and industry as equal partners in the scientific and technical discussions of worldwide testing procedures. ICH brings together experts from the pharmaceutical industry and the regulatory authorities from Europe, Japan and the United States to discuss scientific and technical aspects of product registration for new drugs. ICH addresses Quality, Safety, Efficacy and Multidisciplinary Topics. Of particular interest to a discussion on ethics are the Efficacy Topics, which define standards for conducting clinical studies in human subjects, including Good Clinical Practice (GCP).*

GCP refers to an international ethical and scientific quality standard for designing, conducting, performing, monitoring, auditing, recording, analyzing and reporting of clinical trials that involve participation of human subjects.[iv] The objective of GCP guidelines is to provide a unified standard for

* Other Efficacy Topics include standards for dose response studies, standards for carcinogenicity testing in subjects and clinical safety data management.

the European Union, Japan and the United States to facilitate the mutual acceptance of clinical data by the regulatory authorities in these locations. The guidelines were developed with consideration for the current good clinical practices of the European Union, Japan, the United States, Australia, Canada, the Nordic countries and the World Health Organization.[v]

Based on the GCP guidelines from the ICH, the Food and Drug Administration published *Good Clinical Practice: Consolidated Guidelines* in 1996.[vi] This document describes minimum information to be included in the investigator's brochure together with the essential paperwork needed to permit evaluation of the conduct of a clinical study and the quality of data produced. The FDA requires that the biomedical research it regulates conform to GCP standards as articulated in the FDA regulations. Compliance with GCP provides public assurance that the rights, well-being and confidentiality of trial subjects are protected and clinical data are credible. A few of the GCP guidelines appear in Table 3.

A Sampling of the FDA's "Good Clinical Practice: Consolidated Guidelines"
4.3.2–During and following a subject's participation in a trial, the investigator/institution should ensure that adequate medical care is provided to the subject for any adverse events, including clinically significant laboratory values, related to the trial. The investigator/institution should inform a subject when medical care is needed for intercurrent illness(es) of which the investigator becomes aware.
4.8.7–Before informed consent may be obtained, the investigator, or a person designated by the investigator, should provide the subject, or the subject's legally acceptable representative ample time and opportunity to inquire about details of the trial and to decide whether or not to participate in the trial.
4.11.1–All serious adverse events (SAEs) should be reported immediately to the sponsor except those SAEs that the protocol or other documents (e.g., investigator's brochure) identify as not needing immediate reporting The immediate reports should be followed by detailed, written reports.

Table 3 Source: Good Clinical Practice: Consolidated Guidelines

Ethical Guidelines at the Site Level

In the simplest terms, the intent of ethical guidelines is to protect the study subject from undue harm, to prohibit coercion of potential subjects, to report serious adverse events (SAEs) immediately to the FDA and to ensure that the investigator is trained in good clinical practice. On a daily basis, it would seem that these are largely common sense principles rooted in the ancient concept of "First, do no harm."

But there is more to ethics than treating patients with respect and offering the best care. It means always maintaining the highest ethical standards and training the clinical staff so that they are aware of ethical guidelines and their responsibilities regarding study conduct. It also means reporting known unethical behavior to FDA. All parties with information about misconduct by any clinical professional are encouraged by FDA to report it.[vii] It means turning down a trial that, in your estimation, appears to be unethical. For example, at Palm Beach Research Center, we have walked away from wound studies testing investigational antibiotics because they contained placebo arms. We have turned down studies evaluating use of second-line or third-line drugs that are stronger and associated with more side effects than safer first-line drugs for treatment of the same condition.

FDA has an interest in evaluating ethics at the site level prompted largely by the May 1999 *New York Times* story of a fraudulent Southern California investigator and a companion piece about sponsors enticing investigators with huge sums to enroll patients. Following the media attention garnered by these two stories, the Office of Inspector General (OIG) of the Department of Health and Human Services (HHS) conducted two separate inquiries. The first involved looking at recruitment practices and research sponsored by the drug industry, and the second sought to determine whether there is adequate oversight in place to detect possible fraud by clinical investigators.[viii]

The first inquiry explored use of private doctors in research, and whether this creates conflicts of interest between the doctor's obligations to the patient and his or her responsibilities to the drug company sponsoring the trial. OIG examined use of financial incentives to encourage doctors to accelerate patient recruitment, including payments made for each patient enrolled, and bonuses used to encourage recruitment of the targeted number of patients. The second study examined whether the FDA's authority to disqualify investigators who are either dishonest or who fail to follow procedure is being used in a way that properly protects participants in clinical trials.[ix]

Two final reports issued in June 2000 present the results of these inquiries along with recommendations. The key finding in *Recruiting Human Subjects: Pressures in Industry-Sponsored Clinical Research* highlights an erosion of informed consent driven by the need to accelerate patient recruitment[x] (Table 4). Secondly, there is concern over the compromise of patient confidentiality, and the enrolling of ineligible subjects to meet enrollment targets. The report discusses a survey of 200 IRBs that revealed that generally, IRBs are uncertain of their authority to review certain patient recruitment practices, particularly those that are separate from the investigator-patient relationship.

Erosion of Informed Consent

"The most fundamental concern is that the consent process may be undermined when, under pressure to recruit quickly, for example, investigators misrepresent the true nature of the research or when patients are influenced to participate in research due to their trust in their doctor."

Table 4 Source: Office of Inspector General

The top recommendation of the report is for HHS to provide IRBs with direction regarding oversight of recruitment practices. Specifically, the report calls for HHS to clarify that IRBs have the authority to review certain recruiting practices based on existing federal regulation and to disseminate guidance on what IRBs can address in their review of recruitment practices. Several other recommendations for IRBs are detailed in Table 5.[xi]

Recommendations
Provide IRBs with direction regarding oversight of recruitment practices
Facilitate the development of guidelines for all parties on appropriate recruiting practices
Ensure that IRBs and investigators are adequately educated about human subject protections
Strengthen federal oversight of IRBs

Table 5 Source: Office of Inspector General

Recruiting Human Subjects: Sample Guidelines for Practice[xii] examines a broad base of issues, including recruitment incentives that sponsors give to investigators to boost enrollment; referral fees that nonparticipating physicians receive for referring patients to investigators; conflicts of interest arising from the fact that a patient's physician can have the dual role of also being an investigator in a study for which the physician is recruiting; and the review of confidential medical records by investigators to determine if a patient could qualify for a trial. To conduct the research, OIG gathered information from numerous IRBs, many at academic institutions; and from twenty different medical associations. The participating institutions were asked to provide their guidelines for acceptable patient recruitment and study conduct practices. The purpose of this research was to provide reference points that will stimulate discussion as to what constitutes appropriate recruitment practices and how to develop guidelines that ensure that appropriate practices are adhered to.

Federal Oversight

The June 2000 reports from the Office of Inspector General are part of a larger federal presence that is scrutinizing clinical research. Following these reports and others highlighting pervasive deficiencies at some IRBs, there has been a call to action to improve federal oversight of clinical trials, including detection of fraud committed by investigators. Among the hot-button topics are ethical human subject recruitment, adequacy of informed consent, adherence to good clinical practice and investigators' financial conflicts of interest.

A host of government agencies that report to the HHS are involved in scrutinizing investigator activities such as scientific misconduct, misuse of human and animal research subjects, financial mismanagement and conflict of interest. The offices within HHS that have an investigative function as part of their overall operations are:[xiii]

- **Office of Research Integrity (ORI)**—Handles allegations of scientific misconduct involving HHS-supported research that fits within the definition shown in Table 6.[xiv] To report this type of scientific misconduct, call 301-443-5330.

- **Office of Regulatory Affairs (ORA), Division of Compliance Policy, Bioresearch Monitoring Program (BIMO)**—Investigates allegation of misconduct in regulated research monitored by the FDA. This involves research that is funded both publicly and non-publicly, focusing on human and animal drugs, human biologics, medical devices and food and feed additives. ORA may also take actions related to FDA-regulated research if it is supported by public funds. To report this type of scientific misconduct, call 301-827-0425.

- **Office for Human Research Protections (OHRP)**—Responds to allegations of misuse of human and animal subjects in research supported by HHS. This covers allegations in the area of failure to obtain informed consent from human subjects, mistreatment of human and animal subjects in research, failure to get approval from an IRB or animal care committee and improper care of research animals. To report this type of behavior, call 301-496-7005.

- **Office of Management Assessment (OMA)**—Responsible for reviewing allegation of misuse of funds and grants from the National Institutes of Health (NIH). This includes conflict of interest, improper employee conduct, violations of grant and contract regulations or policy that are not directly tied to misuse of funds. To report this type of behavior, call 301-496-1873.

Definition of Scientific Misconduct

"Fabrication, falsification, plagiarism and other practices that seriously deviate from commonly accepted practices within the scientific community for proposing, conducting, and reporting research. It does not include honest error or honest differences in interpretations or judgments of data."

Table 6 Source: Office of Research Integrity

The level of activity experienced by these offices suggests that today's environment may be more conducive to the reporting of problems, possibly as a result of increased media attention on clinical trials gone awry. The FDA, for example, has traditionally received a small volume of complaints and issued few sanctions against clinical investigators. That changed in 1999 when there was a tenfold increase in the number of complaints filed against investigative sites over the previous year (Figure 1). In 1999, approximately 60% of the complaints targeted the principal investigator or sub-investigator. This number rose to nearly 70% in 2000.[xv]

Stan Woollen, then associate director for bioresearch monitoring, Office of Human Research Trials, within the FDA, said in 2001, "The number of complaints has gone up significantly in the last two years. I can only speculate that it's because of a heightened awareness of clinical trials in general, reflected in media accounts and congressional interest in the trials area. Also, we have actively encouraged sponsors and others to be forthcoming in filing complaints and fulfilling their regulatory responsibilities to us."[xvi] Woollen adds that some complaints are from disgruntled employees but every complaint must be documented and evaluated.[xvii] The FDA assigns inspections to approximately half of all complaints that it receives.

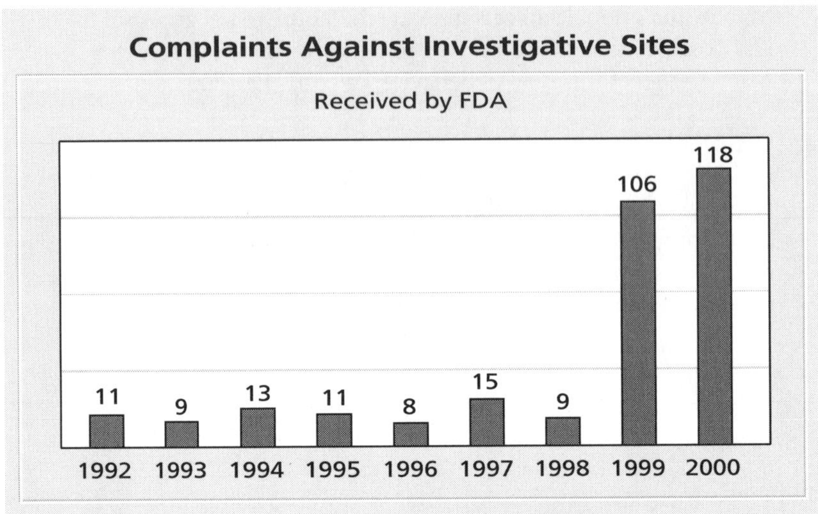

Figure 1 Source: FDA Division of Safety Inspection, CenterWatch

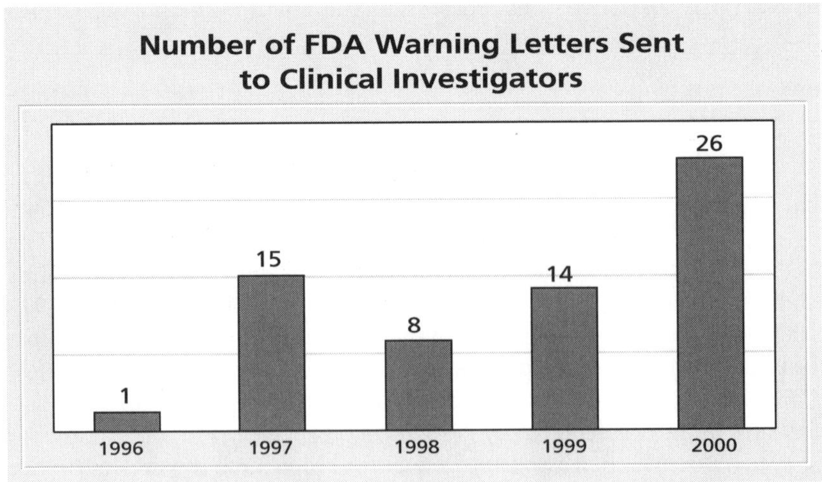

Figure 2 Source: www.fda.gov

The number of FDA warning letters sent to clinical investigators nearly doubled between 1999 and 2000 (Figure 2). This may be in response to a near 30% increase in the number of on-site clinical inspections (Figure 3). Determining the status of these warnings is difficult without examining each case because the FDA does not compile summary updates. The primary areas of investigator deficiencies based on FDA audits and complaints received are: [xviii, xix]

- Protocol non-compliance
- Falsification of data
- Recordkeeping deficiencies
- Poor adverse events reporting
- Poor drug accountability
- Informed consent non-compliance

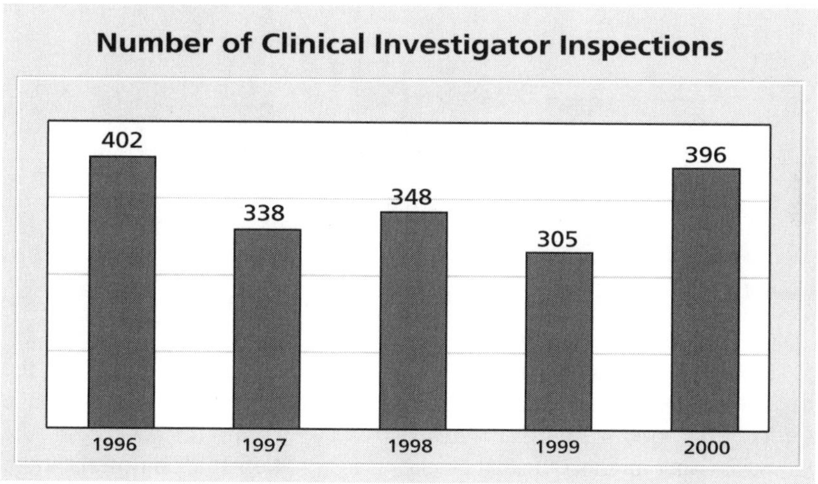

Figure 3 Source: CDER

Overseeing agencies can dispense sanctions beyond the issuance of warning letters. FDA maintains two "black lists" on clinical investigators: the "Debarment List," which names investigators who have been convicted of a felony under the Federal Food, Drug, and Cosmetic Act, and the "Disqualified/Restricted/Assurances List," which cites investigators for various issues of non-compliance (Figure 4). "Disqualified" implies an investigator who is ineligible to receive investigational product. "Restricted" means that an investigator agrees to some restricted use of the investigational product. "Assurances" refers to an investigator who has ensured at a regulatory hearing that performance on future studies with investigational products will comply with regulations. No sanctions are imposed on investigators who have given assurances because of their promise to perform studies in a compliant manner. At the time of this writing, there are 57 investigators on the debarment list and 139 on the disqualified/restricted/assurances list.

The Public Health Service's Office of Research Integrity (ORI) maintains an "Administrative Actions Listing," which names investigators against whom the ORI has imposed sanctions. Currently, there are 35 investigators on that list.[xx]

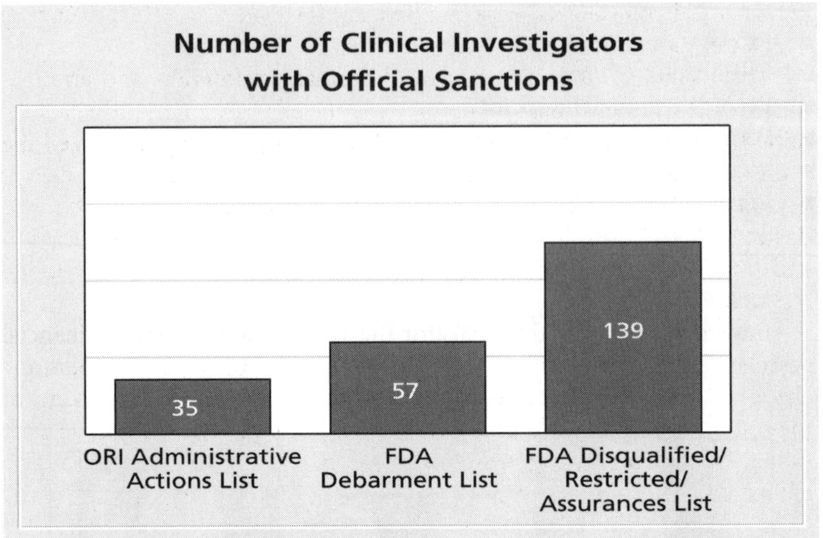

Figure 4 Source: FDA

There are several initiatives within the FDA and HHS to improve the quality and safety of clinical trials. One such example is the formation of the Office for Good Clinical Practice (OGCP), within the Office of the Commissioner and its Office of Science Coordination and Communication, within the FDA. This office replaces the FDA's Office for Human Research Trials, recognizing the distinct roles of the FDA's OGCP from the Department's Office for Human Research Protections (OHRP). The OGCP will continue to work across the Agency and with OHRP to promote the protection of human research participants. In addition, OGCP will work closely with the Centers and Office of Regulatory Affairs to support the quality and integrity of clinical trials and applications submitted to the FDA. OGCP will also work within the FDA and international colleagues to support global harmonization of GCP standards.

Financial Disclosure by Investigators

A major concern regarding investigator conduct is the influence—either perceived or real—that profits have on scientific discovery.[xxi] Because the profit motive could affect the tactics used to recruit and enroll study subjects, as well as on the integrity of the data collected, this subject has been under scrutiny for several years.

During the 1990s, the FDA learned about problematic financial arrangements through published articles, Congressional inquiries, public testimony and comments.[xxii] The result of that effort led to a set of federal regulations known as "Financial Disclosure by Clinical Investigators" or 21 CFR Part 54, which went into effect on February 2, 1999.

These regulations seek to ensure that financial interests and arrangements of clinical investigators that could affect the reliability of data submitted to the FDA are identified and disclosed by the applicant (i.e., the sponsor). This disclosure is required by anyone who submits clinical data as part of an FDA marketing application for any drug, biological product or device and is to include certain information concerning the compensation and financial interests of any clinical investigator involved in conducting research studies for the applicant.

Investigators conducting trials for the sponsors must disclose financial arrangements on disclosure statement forms and must agree to report any changes to their financial disclosure statements if relevant changes occur in the course of the trial or for one year following completion of a clinical trial. (Table 7) Disclosure requirements extend to the spouse and to each dependent child of the investigator.

Required Financial Disclosure Per 21 CFR Part 54
Compensation made to the clinical investigator whose value could be affected by the study outcome.
Proprietary interest, such as a patient, by the investigator in the tested product.
Significant equity interest, i.e., ownership interest, stock options or other financial interest in the sponsor of a study that is ongoing or completed.
Any equity interest that exceeds $50,000 in value in a publicly held sponsor company for which the investigator is conducting studies. The requirement applies to interests held during the time the clinical investigator is carrying out the study and for one year following the completion of the study.
Significant payment by the sponsor of other sorts with a monetary value of more than $25,000, such as grants to fund ongoing research, compensation in the form of equipment or retainers for ongoing consultation or honoraria during the time the clinical investigator is conducting the study and for one year following the completion of the study.

Table 7 Source: Guidance for Industry "Financial Disclosure by Clinical Investigators"

Sponsors submitting marketing applications to the FDA must certify the absence of certain financial interests of clinical investigators on Form FDA 3454 and disclose those financial interests on Form FDA 3455. The FDA may refuse to file any market applications that do not include these properly completed forms or a certification by the applicant that it has acted with due diligence to obtain the information but has been unable to do so and why.[xxiii]

The goal of the regulations is to eliminate financial arrangements that could encourage clinical investigators to bias the results of their clinical trials. According to Part 54.1(b), "FDA may consider clinical studies inadequate and the data inadequate if, among other things, appropriate steps have not been taken in the design, conduct reporting, and analysis of the studies to minimize bias."

While many clinicians, sponsors and CROs support the concept of financial disclosure, implementing the ruling remains difficult because the FDA has not established clear guidelines for reviewing financial disclosures. Specifically, the FDA has identified only general actions it can take to handle the discovery that a significant financial interest exists between an investigator—or that of the investigator's immediate family—and the sponsor. The March 2001 FDA guidance entitled, *Financial Disclosure by Clinical Investigators, a Guidance for Industry*[xxiv] states, "If FDA determines that the financial interests of any clinical investigator raise a serious question about the integrity of the data, FDA will take action it deems necessary to ensure the reliability of the data." Actions are listed in Table 8, but specific action is left to the discretion of the FDA reviewer.

FDA Actions That Can Be Taken if There is a Question About Data Integrity Linked to Financial Interests of Any Clinical Investigator

Initiate agency audits of the data derived from the clinical investigator in question.
Request that the applicant submit further analyses of the data.
Request that the applicant conduct additional independent studies to confirm the results of the questioned study.
Refuse to treat the covered clinical study as providing data that can be the basis for an agency action.

Table 8 Source: Guidance for Industry "Financial Disclosure by Clinical Investigators"

Other problems stem from the fact that a volatile stock market can change the value of a holding almost daily. According to the FDA guidance, an investigator is to report an equity interest in a publicly traded sponsor company once the value of the holding exceeds the $50,000 threshold. FDA does not expect the investigator to report when the equity interest fluctuates below the $50,000 threshold.[xxv] In addition, the FDA does not see the financial disclosure information of each investigator until the applicant makes a submission. The close monitoring of the investigator's need to disclose is done by the sponsor who according to the regulations, is to be in communication with investigators on this issue.[xxvi] The sponsor is required to keep these records for a period of two years after the date of approval of the application.[xxvii]

The inadequacies of federal regulations governing conflicts of interest has caught the attention of the Senate, which asked the General Accounting Office (GAO) to compile a report on the subject. The GAO issued its report in November 2001 and found federal regulations lacking. One of the most serious limitations, aside from the vagueness of the regulations themselves, is that FDA regulations are not directly linked to the regulations on human subjects protection. The result is that "financial interest information may not necessarily be conveyed to institutional review boards for consideration when they review research proposals for risks to human subjects." In addition, there are two sets of federal regulations—Public Health Service (PHS) regulations, which cover federally funded research, and FDA regulations, which cover privately funded and federally regulated research. The two sets of regulations differ in two areas: "when they require review of investigators' financial disclosures, and in the amounts of their disclosure thresholds." According to PHS regulations, institutions must report financial conflicts of interest on the part of investigators to PHS before research funds are spent. According to FDA regulations, a sponsor only submits that information to FDA after the research has been completed. Both sets of regulations are vague in terms of what constitutes a conflict of interest and how it should be managed.

GAO recommended in its report that the Department of Health and Human Services (HHS) "develop specific guidance or regulations to address institutional financial conflicts of interest." HHS agreed with these recommendations in its comments on a draft of this report.

In Review

There is strong evidence that investigators need to be trained in Good Clinical Practice, guidelines that incorporate a strong ethics component. Although clinical trials have been conducted for centuries, the definition of ethical conduct in clinical trials has been codified through several key documents developed within the past fifty years. Starting in 1947 with the Nuremberg Code, moving to the Declaration of Helsinki adopted by the World Medical Association in 1964, then to the 1979 publishing of the Belmont Report in the

Federal Register, and ending with good clinical practice standards outlines by the International Conference on Harmonization (ICH), there is a vast array of guidelines that every investigator needs to know. The core of these documents focuses on respect for volunteers, protecting them from undue harm and obtaining of informed consent in a non-coercive manner.

Prompted by headline-grabbing stories of wildly fraudulent investigators and multiple GCP violations at leading research institutions, several offices within HHS have been improving oversight of clinical trials at the site level. These offices within the Department, such as the Office of Research Integrity, Office of Regulatory Affairs, Office for Human Research Protections and Office of Management Assessment, are responsible for handling complaints and conducting investigations. The FDA, an HHS agency, historically saw few complaints, but in 1999, experienced a tenfold increase in the number of complaints filed against investigative sites as compared to 1998. The 2000 figures showed an 11% rise in the number of complaints over the previous year. In both years, the majority of complaints were leveled against the principal investigator or sub-investigator.

Numbers such as these may suggest a new awareness of the problem, a greater willingness to report it and/or an influx of untrained investigators. And every complaint does not necessarily mean there is a problem. Violations, if they exist, might be rather minor, requiring no action or voluntary action. Possible offenders are more likely to be operating out of ignorance of their responsibilities rather than malice. Those who are committing felony fraud are going to be more closely scrutinized, and risk being debarred from further clinical research activity, or may face other less punitive sanctions.

At the site level, maintaining the highest ethical standards by embracing GCP concepts is the best way to operate. In order to achieve this, the clinical staff must be trained so they are aware of the standards, and they must also follow common sense rules such as walking away from studies that appear inappropriate or reporting known fraudulent or unethical behavior. The goal is to raise the bar, enabling study volunteers to participate in studies conducted in an overall safe and ethical environment.

The regulations surrounding financial disclosure are vague at best and have caught the attention of many relevent authorities in Washington. New, specific guidelines should be forthcoming in the near future. In the meantime, it is better to err on the side of caution.

References

[i] The Nuremberg Code, 1947, *www.cirp.org/library/ethics/nuremberg*, accessed September 10, 2001.

[ii] The Declaration of Helsinki, *www.wma.net/e/policy/17-c_e.html*, accessed September 10, 2001.

[iii] Belmont Report, *http://ohsr.od.nih.gov/mpa/belmont.php3*, accessed September 11, 2001. The Belmont Report was named for the

Belmont Conference Center at the Smithsonian Institute where the Commission met.

[iv] *www.fda.gov/oc/gcp*, accessed September 20, 2001.

[v] ICH Harmonised Tripartite Guideline: Guideline for Good Clinical Practice, Introduction, 1996, *www.ifpma.org/pdfifpma/e6.pdf*, accessed September 11, 2001.

[vi] Good Clinical Practice: Consolidated Guidelines, *www.fda.gov/cder/guidance/959fnl.pdf*, accessed September 12, 2001.

[vii] Patient Misuse and Investigator Fraud in Clinical Trials: What Can Be Done? *www.fda.gov/cder/present/dia-62000/woolen1/sld058.htm*, accessed September 20, 2001.

[viii] *A Guide to Patient Recruitment*, Diana Anderson, CenterWatch, 2001, pp. 19-21.

[ix] "U.S. Officials are Examining Clinical Trials," *The New York Times*, Kurt Eichenwald, July 14, 1999.

[x] Recruiting Human Subjects: Pressures in Industry-Sponsored Clinical Research, Office of Inspector General, *www.hhs.gov/oig/oei/reports/a459.pdf*, June 2000.

[xi] Ibid., pp. 4-5.

[xii] Recruiting Human Subjects: Sample Guidelines for Practice, Office of Inspector General, *www.hhs.gov/oig/oei/reports/a458.pdf*, June 2000.

[xiii] *http://ori.dhhs.gov/html/about/abuse.asp*, accessed September 13, 2001.

[xiv] *http://ori.dhhs.gov*, accessed April 11, 2001.

[xv] "FDA Complaints Against Investigative Sites Still Rising," *CenterWatch*, June 2001, Vol. 8, Issue 6, Valerie Gamache, p. 12.

[xvi] "Clinical Research in Transition," *The Monitor*, Summer 2001, Vol. 15, Issue 2, Jim Maloy et al., p. 26.

[xvii] Op. cit., *CenterWatch*, p. 5.

[xviii] Patient Misuse and Investigator Fraud in Clinical Trials: What Can be Done? *http://www.fda.gov/cder/present/dia-62000/woolen1/index.htm*, accessed September 15, 2001.

[xix] "FDA Complaints Against Investigative Sites Still Rising," *CenterWatch*, June 2001, Vol. 8, Issue 6, Valerie Gamache, p. 12.

[xx] *http://www.fdalgov/ora/compliance_ref*, accessed September 13, 2001.

[xxi] "Investigator Scrutiny and Certification," ACRP White Paper 2001, *The Monitor*, The Association of Clinical Research Professionals, James W. Maloy et al, Summer 2001, Vol. 15, Issue 2, p. 28.

[xxii] "Financial Disclosure by Clinical Investigators, A Guidance for Industry," March 2001, www.fda.gov/cder.

[xxiii] 21 Code of Federal Regulations (CFR) Part 54.4(3)c.

[xxiv] "Financial Disclosure by Clinical Investigators, A Guidance for Industry," March 2001, www.fda.gov/cder.

[xxv] Ibid.

[xxvi] 21 Code of Federal Regulations (CFR) Part 54.4.

[xxvii] 21 Code of Federal Regulations (CFR) Part 54.6(b)

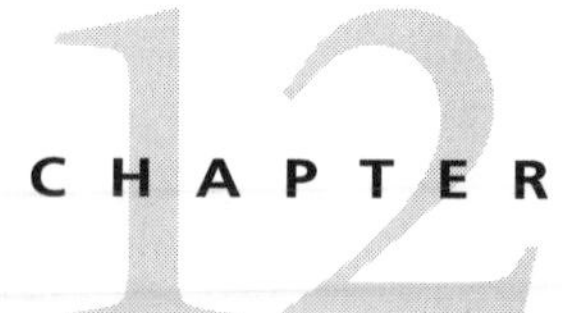

Selling Your Site

- What Is Your Site Worth?
- Asset Approach
- Market Data or Comparables Approach
- Structuring the Deal
- The Market for Selling Your Site
- To Whom Should You Sell?
- It's an Emotional Decision

It's a constant struggle. Cash flow shortages, paperwork overload, personnel problems, broken air conditioning, severe weather. These are problems that could plague any business. But when the product of that business is quality data generated from human research subjects, there seems to be a heightened level of stress.

Some site owners love the clinical trials business and thrive on the daily stresses and challenges associated with it. Others who also love clinical research yearn to escape the constant headaches that stem from management and operations issues. They would prefer to focus on seeing patients, leaving others to handle the thousands of administrative details. This is one group of site owners who, once they have achieved a level of growth, may contemplate selling the site. A survey of owners who had sold their sites to site management organizations (SMOs) gave several more reasons for selling:[i]

- It represents an approach to survival—to better address intensifying market competition for clinical grants.

- It offers an opportunity to refine and improve site operations and add marketing, sales and administrative infrastructure.
- It may offer more growth, i.e., joining an SMO carries the promise of higher clinical study volume.
- It is an important exit strategy for soon-to-be-retiring investigators.

Whatever the reason for considering selling the site, there are as many ways to structure deals as there are people putting them together. Although the details vary from deal to deal, there are several basic issues surrounding the sale of a clinical site (Table 1). Perhaps the most significant concern is whether the owner and top managers plan to stay at the site once it is sold. Because a site's chief asset is its staff and the experience they bring to clinical research trials, a potential buyer generally to wants them to remain at the site, under contract, for at least a few years. A facility without the principal investigator and staff is little more than office space.

Key Factors to Consider When Planning to Sell Your Site
Deciding whether the owner and medical director plan to remain at the site
Determining what the site is worth
Researching the track record, caliber and reputation of potential buyers

Table 1

A second major issue is placing a dollar value on the site. Prospective buyers and sellers use various formulae to arrive at an asking or bidding price for the site. Thirdly, a prospective seller who plans to remain at the site after it is sold needs to explore the track record of potential buyers to determine their success rate and their commitment to operating the site in an ethical and profitable manner. Like most industries, the clinical trials world is small, so news of affiliating with either competent or unscrupulous operators will spread quickly.

What Is Your Site Worth?

Many factors figure into the valuation of a site. On the number-crunching side, there's the history of gross and net profits from the past few years, value and age of outstanding receivables, number of studies booked for the near future, and cost of fixed and variable expenses. On the intangible side of the equation, there's the owner's interest in remaining at the site after the sale and his or her motivation for selling; the caliber of the staff, the perceived value of the therapeutic specialties offered by the site, the condition of the standard operating procedures (SOPs) and the status of the market for outsourcing of studies. Determining the investigative site's fair market value is the art and science of balancing numbers with non-numerical factors. One business appraised at $400,000 may sell for $300,000, while another business equally appraised may sell for $500,000. The difference in selling price reflects various factors unique to each situation.

From a numbers perspective, there are three standard methods for valuing businesses:[ii]

- Earnings approach
- Asset approach
- Market Data or Comparables approach

Each approach gives a different vantage point to the appraiser, accountant, business broker or investment firm responsible for establishing a range of value. For this reason, professionals who value a business tend to use more than one valuation method to arrive at a balanced figure. It is also worth mentioning that the term "earnings" is often used loosely but actually has various definitions such as pre-tax profit; earnings before interest, taxes, depreciation and amortization (EBITDA); after-tax profit; operating profit, etc. Appraisers often use pre-tax earnings because after-tax figures are subject to many manipulations designed to reduce income tax liability.[iii]

It is not within the scope of this book to provide detailed analyses of each method as there are entire books dedicated to this subject. Instead, what follows is a brief overview of key approaches and definitions and their application to the clinical trials business.

The Earnings approach is based on the earnings of the business and embraces the fundamental reason for buying a business: to receive the company's stream of profits.[iv] The earnings approach refers to a collection of various methods (Table 2), but one that has application for the clinical trials industry is Discounted Future Earnings. Valuation is started by adding together the anticipated annual earnings for the next few years. For example, if a site is expected to have earnings of $20,000 in each of the next five years, showing flat growth, the expected earnings stream is $100,000. If the buyer anticipates the earnings to grow at a specific rate, based on current and historic earnings, he or she factors in that growth rate. In addition to the earnings growth rate, the buyer will have a desired rate of return based on how risky he or she perceives the business to be.

Besides adding together the future income stream, the discounted future earnings method includes:

- Determining the present value of this income stream
- Estimating the value of the business at the end of the ownership period
- Adding these two values together

Determining the present value of the income stream is one of the most basic elements of valuing a business. Establishing present value can be explained by the following simple example.

Various Earnings Approaches to Valuing a Business
Discounted Future Earnings
Discounted Future Cash Flow
Simple Price/Earnings (P/E) Ratios
Capitalized Earnings

Table 2 Source: Wright, 1990

> An investigative site expects to have earnings of $100,000 over the next five years, earned equally as $20,000 per year. A buyer interested in purchasing the site is developing an offer and wants to determine the present value of that $100,000. In making his calculations, he factors in a 10% rate of return on his investment. Using the 10% rate of return, known as the "discount factor," there is the following calculation:*

Present Value (PV) of $20,000 to be received in one year =	$18,181.80
PV of $20,000 to be received in two years =	16,529.00
PV of $20,000 to be received in three years =	15,026.20
PV of $20,000 to be received in four years =	13,660.20
PV of $20,000 to be received in five years =	12,418.40
Total:	$75,815.60

As this example illustrates, if the buyer pays $75,815.60 to the seller today, and receives $100,000 at the end of five years, the buyer will have received his required 10% return on investment.

In addition to computing the present value on the five-year income stream, the buyer often estimates the value of the business at the end of an ownership period, which in this case is five years. Doing a thorough analysis

* Factors are: 1 year = 0.90909; 2 years = 0.82645; 3 years = 0.75131; 4 years = 0.68301; 5 years = 0.62092.

of the "terminal value" is beyond the scope of this chapter, but it is possible to estimate "terminal value" by using a multiple derived from a ratio known as price/earnings per share, or P/E.

For publicly traded companies, P/E is the relationship of a company's stock price to its earnings per share. So, a company whose stock sells for $10/share and has earnings of $1/share has a P/E of 10. For small, privately held businesses, such as travel agencies, restaurants, retail businesses, etc., P/E multiples have been established from a variety of factors such as degree of risk and length of time the company has been in business (Table 3).[v] Professional practices are often assigned a P/E range of 1 to 5.[vi] Although there are general P/E ratios for various industries, each business is unique, so the P/E ratio should be developed for each transaction. Using a predetermined P/E ratio is too simplistic to provide a meaningful valuation of a specific business, and serves more as a thumbnail sketch or approximation of value.

Factors that Figure into Price/Earnings Multiplier
Degree of risk
Length of time in business
Length of time current owner has owned the business
Owner's motivation for selling
Profitability
Business location
Growth history
Competition
Entry barriers
Future market for the industry
Customer base
Information systems infrastructure

Table 3 Source: Snowden, 1993

When estimating value through the use of P/E, it is wise to make fairly conservative assumptions because no one can predict market conditions and interest rates five years into the future. Using a conservative P/E ratio of

3, the following calculation can be made to determine a rough estimate of terminal value:

P/E of 3 x $12,418.40 (amount to be received in five years in example above) = $37,255.20

The business is worth roughly:

Discounted earnings:	$75,815.60
Terminal value:	+ 37,255.20
Approximate value of business:	$113,070.80

The Discounted Cash Flow Method is similar to the Discounted Future Earnings Method except the company's free cash flow is used instead of earnings to compute net present value. Free cash flow refers to the amount of cash left after allowing for necessary investment in new assets such as equipment and leasehold improvements.[vii]

The Capitalized Earnings Method[viii] develops the business valuation by using the actual adjusted earnings stream of the business from the past few years plus the rate of return that the buyer requires in order to invest in this business. The purpose of this method is to determine the true earnings of the company in a typical operating year. It places no value on equipment and fixed assets. The actual earnings stream is adjusted for unusually large revenues or expenses that occurred in the past year or two because they cannot reasonably be expected to reoccur in the near future. For example, if a site landed one unusually large contract two years ago, a potential buyer cannot expect to procure others of that size on a regular basis. For this reason, a site with $500,000 in adjusted earnings over the past three years of $100,000, $150,000, and $250,000 might be a safer bet than a site with equal adjusted earnings earned as $50,000, $350,000, and $100,000. Similarly, a site that earned its profits from ten studies last year may be worth more than one that made 80% of profits from one study.

Once the earnings stream is adjusted for unusual expenses and/or revenues the buyer will develop a multiplier known as the capitalization rate. Different than a P/E ratio, the "cap rate" determines the rate of return that an investor expects to get on an investment of this type. The cap rate reflects current earnings and no future earnings. The Build-Up Method is one way to compute the cap rate[ix] and is shown in the following example:

Annual yield on risk-free Treasury notes:	5%
Return for business ownership risk:	12%
Return for risk of small business:	3%
Minus long-term annual growth rate:	(5%)
Cap Rate:	15%

The cap rate is converted into a multiplier by dividing it into 100%. Thus, a cap rate of 15% would yield a multiplier of 6.67. With this method, the business with average adjusted earnings of $500,000 over three years, equaling $166,667 per year, would be valued as follows:

Average adjusted earnings per year:	$166,667
Cap rate multiplier:	x 6.67
Approximate value of the business:	$1,111,668.89

This is a good method to use in a stable industry. It is less reliable in a growing industry because it does not consider future earnings potential. When using this method in a growing industry, last year's revenues may be weighted more heavily than those that are three or four years old.

Asset Approach

It is obvious that every business has assets it uses to operate. There is equipment unique to that business, office furniture and supplies and leasehold improvements. In the case of a clinical research site, there are likely to be pieces of medical equipment and possibly lab supplies. For the purposes of valuation, assets are usually viewed at their market value or replacement value instead of their accounting value as shown on the company's books. Replacement value is frequently higher than book value if the accountant has used accelerated depreciation expenses to reduce the tax burden.[x] If this is the case, the owner's equity is worth more than the amount shown on the books.

This method—known as adjusted book value, adjusted balance sheet, or net tangible asset value—has little application to clinical research because it places a heavy emphasis on replacement value of plant and equipment, appreciation of land and other real estate and understated or overstated inventories due to accounting method. Clinical research is a very labor-intensive business, and a buyer is essentially interested in the staff's reputation and ability to conduct clinical trials. The equipment is secondary in importance.

Market Data or Comparables Approach

In theory, the best way to value your site is to find other sites like yours that have sold recently, and look up their sale prices and the factors leading to the sale price. Valuing companies in this way is known as the Market Data or Comparables Approach. When publicly traded companies are involved, information about standard ratios such as price/earnings, price/book and price/revenue are publicly available. For small, privately held investigative sites, however, finding information about sales of comparable publicly traded companies can be challenging because most, if not all, of the players are also privately held. Details generally are not disclosed, and the smaller the company, the less likely that the appraiser will be able to find one or more good comparables, public or private.[xi]

This method involves finding out:

- Annual gross revenue
- Earnings
- Assets
- Cash flow

With this information, a simplistic valuation can be determined as follows:

> An investigative site was recently sold for $100,000. If gross revenues were $150,000 and earnings were $18,000, the business sold for 0.67 times revenues and 5.6 times earnings.

If any piece of the information is unavailable, appraisers would be likely to use other approaches or a combination of approaches to avoid making erroneous valuations. For example, if two sites each had pre-tax earnings last year of $16,000, but their annual gross revenues are unknown, it would not make sense to use this method of valuation. Similarly, if there is no information about unusual expenses or revenues, it is difficult to make a meaningful valuation. The Market Data approach is better used for valuing publicly traded companies.

Structuring the Deal

Selling a research site is all about the seller negotiating an acceptable buyout package with the buyer who expects to use the site to grow the earnings stream through the conduct of clinical research. The first step in creating the offer is for the buyer to determine the value of the site. Placing a value on the site requires the use of various accounting methods. Eric Hayashi, vice president of corporate development at Radiant Research, explains that the company generally uses three approaches:

- Discounted Cash Flow (DCF) analysis
- Earnings before interest, taxes, depreciation and amortization (EBITDA)
- Competition

By combining the results of these methods, Radiant "triangulates in" on a value that it uses to formulate an offer. The DCF analysis enables the buyer to determine the present value of projected cash flow based on anticipated growth rates of earnings and factors in the desired rate of return or "discount factor." This analysis is critical because the company believes that the true value of the site stems from its ability to generate future cash flow. Hayashi says that developing a realistic cash flow projection depends on the age of the site's historical performance and study pipeline. "A clinic that has consistently produced cash flow of $500,000 annually for each of the past five years has less risk than a newer site that has produced less cash flow, so our acceptable rate of return may be lower for the older site. The newer site has more risk but may have greater prospects for growth. For this reason, the older site may not necessarily earn a higher valuation than the newer site," comments Hayashi.

Next, Radiant computes EBITDA and compares that to gross revenues. For example, if Site #1 has gross revenues of $2 million and earnings of $300,000 before interest, taxes, depreciation and amortization, this suggests a level of expenses and operational efficiencies different from Site #2 with EBITDA of $200,000 on the same gross revenues. It also suggests that Site #1 may have cut staff inappropriately to improve the bottom line, or may have had a lucky year with one study representing 50% of revenues. Site #2 may have lower EBITDA because it is overloaded with expenses in an effort to decrease the tax burden. For example, inflated salaries, leases for luxury cars, discretionary cash, country club dues and boat slip fees that are listed as business expenses may have served to reduce Site #2's earnings.

In a case such as this, the buyer will want to look at EBITDA for the trailing two or three years to determine if Site #1 had a positive blip last year but was otherwise erratic in earnings, whereas Site #2 was actually the more "Steady Eddie" in terms of earnings consistency. Radiant also compares acquisition candidates' financials relative to its existing sites and seeks to understand variances and to identify areas where it could improve a sites' performance (i.e., decrease in marketing costs). Because of the many variables involved, using EBITDA in conjunction with other valuation methods can be particularly helpful.

The third piece of Radiant's evaluation is to consider the impact that competitive bids for the site have on its offer. This is where non-financial issues come into play. A competitive bidder who believes that the prospective site has higher earnings growth potential would logically make a higher offer more than another competitor who projects more modest growth. Obviously, this will drive up the offer price.

Lee Palles, CEO of nTouch Research Corporation, says his company also uses a combination of financial and non-financial methods to determine valuation. The company looks at some classic financial benchmarks such as multiples of projected cash flow and discounted earnings and considers the immediate backlog of business. Next, the company evaluates subjective criteria such as understanding the culture of the site, the caliber of the staff and the therapeutic expertise offered by the site.

Placing an intangible value on the clinical staff is certainly essential. Without a doubt, the key assets of a site are the people who perform the work. This includes experienced investigators and trained coordinators who are able to procure studies because of their proven expertise and their contacts with sponsors. The value assigned to good will reflects the staff's reputation and their willingness to stay and perform at the same high level of motivation for a new owner.

Because so much of the site's identity is tied up in the principal investigator and staff, the buyer's offer often requires the principal investigator to stay for a reasonable period of time to encourage a smooth transition. This assumes that the buyer sees this investigator as someone who will be able to accept direction from the new owner and is willing to relinquish the reins as chief decision maker.

If the principal investigator agrees to stay after the sale, at least for several years, the site is likely to be worth more than one whose investigator plans to retire and exit the business shortly thereafter. Hayashi says, "We typically do not allow a very short employment period for the principal investigator. We have declined investigator-owner offers where the investigator simply wants to sell his or her business. Part of our typical deal is the physician signs a five year employment agreement. Then we can mutually develop a transition period for the investigator to help cultivate a new medical director for the site." Palles adds, "The investigator who wants to retire after the sale creates a very difficult set of circumstances because once he or she leaves, the business's value is greatly diminished. For a research site, the only loyalty is the sponsor who has a history with the principal investigator and a knowledge of his or her expertise. Without that, the buyer of such a business is taking quite a risk and that is usually reflected in the pricing of the site."

It is important to create incentives so the principal investigator who stays is motivated to perform at the same high level as before the sale. An investigator who stays after the sale but suddenly starts performing like a disinterested employee will have obvious negative impact on the site. To avoid this, the buyer and seller may negotiate some part of the package to include remuneration tied to site performance. This takes the form of cash, percentage of profits or stock options. For example, a portion of the payout may be paid in cash in years 1 and 2 after the sale, the amount being tied to percentage increase in earnings before interest, taxes, depreciation and amortization (EBITDA). Another method is to pay the investigator a continuing percentage of the profits. A third option is to offer equity or company stock. Obviously, the better the stock performs, the greater the benefit to the seller who is at least partially responsible for the stock performance.

Accepting stock is a gamble. At the time of this writing, buyers are generally privately held concerns with their own stock. If buyers go public, there could be a discounted offer price available to the seller, but there is no way to predict the performance of that stock three to five years in advance. Obviously, if the stock is successful, the seller's buyout deal will have an increased value. The reverse can also happen.

The details of each deal are different, reflecting the seller's motivations and interest in staying after the sale. For example, two sites that are going to be sold at $1 million each can have vastly different terms. If the principal investigator plans to stay at the site, she might accept a deal from a site management organization (SMO) that includes one-third cash up front, one-third in a four-year note and one-third in a convertible note that converts into the SMO's equity (at a discounted price) at the owner's option. If the owner chooses not to convert, the balance is paid out in cash at predetermined intervals.

Another owner who wants more cash up front may opt for a deal that pays 40% cash up front, 30% in a five-year note with an interest rate linked to site performance and 30% in a convertible note. Other owners may want to defer cash because of tax consequences.

Before accepting an offer from the seller, we advise visiting a trusted tax advisor to learn the tax implications of the deal.

The Market for Selling Your Site

The late 1990s was somewhat of a frenetic period for acquisition of individual sites. They were being acquired at a rapid pace largely by site management organizations (SMOs) as the young industry began consolidating. The trend, peaking in 1998, started slowing by 2000, dropping to only four acquired individual sites (Figure 1).[**,xii] At the time of this writing, third quarter 2001, only two investigative sites had been purchased year-to-date. The mood of the industry suggests that the pace has slowed substantially and is expected to stay slow through the first few years of the new millennium.

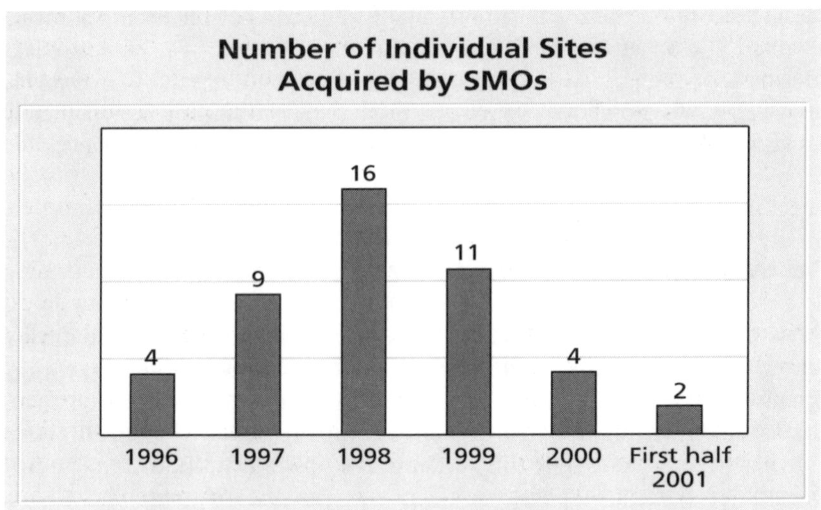

Figure 1 Source: CenterWatch

** Overall figures for 2000 were boosted, however, by two major SMO purchases. Radiant Research bought 20 sites from the HillTop Research network, and nTouch Research's purchase of Health Advance Institute increased its presence by seven sites.

As explained in Chapter 9, several reasons have been cited for the slowdown. One reason may be that large independent sites that wanted to be acquired have already done so. The remaining pool of sites interested in being acquired may be performing lower numbers of clinical trials annually and may have less experience than their predecessors.[xiii] Additionally, SMOs have had a challenging time integrating their acquisitions into their corporate structures, in terms of improving site profitability and encouraging entrepreneurial investigators to conform to corporate policy. Because many of the acquired sites were already operating frugally prior to acquisition, there was a limited amount of additional profitability left to squeeze out of them. Finally, some SMOs have had difficulty with sponsors accepting the SMO concept. A 1999 survey of 25 sponsors showed that on average, SMOs contribute three sites per multi-center trial, not enough to impact study startup and patient recruitment significantly.[xiv]

This lack of acceptance of the concept and a failure to deliver on promises has caused a number of SMOs to exit the business. Consequently, the field is left with fewer buyers. Those who are left are still considering acquisitions, but may be more focused on integrating acquisitions they have already made. The reduction in the number of buyers and their increased attention to integration of sites already acquired is bound to lead to lower site valuations. Hayashi of Radiant Research says, "My sense is that the valuations may have gone down. I think acquisitions will continue to be quite slow over the next few years."

That's not to say that there won't be ready, willing and able buyers. A basic tenet of business is that anything of value will be able to find a buyer. Perhaps the buyer will be someone who wants to enter the clinical trials business, or someone who owns one site but wants to expand or possibly a small SMO. As more investigative sites reach that critical $1 million in annual grant revenue, more of them may become potential acquisition targets.

To Whom Should You Sell?

Now that your site is approaching $2 million in gross revenues, you dream about selling it to some worthy buyer who sees you as a partner, and who plans to expand gross revenues 30% annually using a combination of smart management techniques, well-organized company-wide SOPs and attractive financial incentives. While this certainly is a possibility, finding a high-caliber buyer doesn't happen by accident. It takes research, observation and common sense. It takes deciding if you would be happier becoming part of a small network, a large, national SMO with centralized functions and corporate structure, or simply retiring. Once prospective buyers start materializing, it behooves the seller to check the creditworthiness of each buyer and its reputation for follow-through on promises.

During the late 1990s, when the acquisition trend was at its peak, Palm Beach Research Centers (PBRC) had some very generous offers, several from companies that are no longer in business. Our ability to avoid risky offers had less to do with any untapped talent for predicting the future than with a gut reaction that made us hesitate. In addition, we were not truly interested in selling.

The exercise was not completely without benefit, however. Having been approached by various suitors did open our eyes to the fact that some buyers are obviously more reliable and respectable than others. On several occasions, potential buyers made sophisticated and impressive sales presentations, explaining how their organizations could help PBRC increase revenues, reduce administrative and regulatory burden and facilitate patient recruitment through a centralized effort. There were promises to follow up with phone calls and letters to confirm the statements made during the presentation, and to set dates for the next meeting. In several cases those phone calls and letters never materialized. In other instances, those calls were three to four weeks late. Sometimes, we placed telephone calls that were never returned. This poor follow-up should raise obvious red flags for a seller, especially one planning to become an employee of the site after the sale. Can the seller trust his or her company and future livelihood to a buyer who is too disorganized or disinterested to keep a promise to make a simple telephone call?

According to a 2000 CenterWatch survey of twenty sites acquired by SMOs, results of those acquisitions have been quite mixed.[xv] All twenty of the sites had been acquired more than two years prior to the survey. Smaller sites were generally happier with the outcome of the acquisition than were larger sites. This difference may stem from the fact that smaller sites, by nature, have less infrastructure, so they stand to benefit substantially from the additional administrative, regulatory and business development support. Some larger sites reported that they did not grow as expected, and that the SMO could not turn around the regulatory, quality assurance, contracting and budgeting functions as quickly as the site could. Some comments from smaller and larger sites appear in Table 4.

There are reputable organizations purchasing sites, resulting in satisfied administrators and investigators. Carlos DuJovne, M.D., Medical Director at Radiant Research's Kansas City site says that his site has become more successful since its acquisition in 1998. It was a two-year-old site with an annual earnings growth rate of 20% prior to acquisition, moving to 50% following the acquisition. DuJovne says, "I consider myself to be in a partnership with Radiant. The company has a great deal of respect for the independent thinking of the investigator and does not create a barrier between the investigator and the sponsor … I have more time to dedicate to medical issues because I leave the administrative and supervisory duties to Radiant."

It's an Emotional Decision

Selling is more than a financial transaction for most sellers. It is also an emotional decision. Watching someone else take ownership and become the key decision maker at a site that the seller grew from scratch would be tough for most people, but this is a natural progression when selling the site is the key exit strategy. Because some investigators wrestle with relinquishing control, they may react in several ways. Some may actually end up working harder for someone else than they did for themselves to earn the incentives built into the contract, and to prove that the site is a worthwhile entity. They may also want

Perceptions of Small and Large Sites About Their Acquisition by SMOs

Some Perceptions of Small Sites	Some Perceptions of Larger Sites
"We've lost autonomy, but at the same time, we've received a lot in return for that. Some of the decision making about where the business is heading, the hiring and firing of people, getting equipment, etc., that's all handled by administration. If problems come up, there are now people to handle it—personnel managers, information systems people running our computer network ...."	"We have not grown when that was the promise. We have had to take back a number of functions: regulatory affairs, quality assurance and contracting and budgeting because our SMO was taking too long."
"I would say that our SMO has met 90% of our expectations."	"Hindsight is 20/20; I've lost equity ... I've lost efficiency."
"I think the contract process is slow, but because it's done centrally, we're smarter and we don't get burned on contracts as much as we used to ... Maintaining cash flow was a major problem for us. Our SMO helped us solve that problem."	"We were promised a lot of new business, but it didn't really pan out for us. There is a lot of seller's remorse for me."

Table 4

Source: CenterWatch

to prove that both parties made the right decision. Others may sabotage the effort by slacking off if they feel a sense of remorse, irritation at watching the buyer take the site in new directions or frustration due to broken promises.

To minimize this result, it cannot be stressed enough that the seller needs to investigate the buyer. Do the required homework which means meet the management team—several times—evaluate the buyer's financial status and the caliber of its strategic plan for the site, the quality of its SOPs, the size of its business development staff and the ability of its regulatory department to turn around documents quickly. Also, speak to others who have been acquired by the same company or have at least done business with it. Get referrals for competent and experienced appraisers, investment bankers, accountants or lawyers to help you value your business. Those with at least some experience in the clinical trials industry are preferred. Do as much research on the buyer as the buyer is doing on the seller. This is particularly important because buyers of clinical sites are generally privately held concerns, meaning that financial information is not publicly available.

The best deals are win/win situations in which the seller becomes a partner with the buyer in equity, in practice and in spirit. Finding this match can be more difficult in today's market, which is slower than the one seen in the late 1990s, especially because there are fewer SMOs around. The remaining ones may be more focused on boosting the profitability of the sites they have already acquired and integrating them into the corporate mold. Nevertheless, there will always be a market for a well-run, profitable site with a well-trained, ethical staff.

References

[i] "A Bitter Pill for SMOs," *CenterWatch*, September 2000, Vol. 7, Issue 9, CenterWatch Editorial, p. 10.

[ii] *What is a Business Worth.* Jeffrey P. Wright, E.V.S. Publications, 1990, p. 3.

[iii] Ibid., p. 15.

[iv] Ibid., pp. 9-25.

[v] Ibid., pp. 146-147.

[vi] *The Complete Guide to Buying a Business*, Robert W. Snowden, American Management Association, 1993, pp. 150-151.

[vii] *What is a Business Worth.* Jeffrey P. Wright, E.V.S. Publications, 1990, pp. 24-25.

[viii] Ibid., pp. 15-19.

[ix] Ibid., p. 17.

[x] Ibid., p. 27.

[xi] *The Valuation of Privately-Held Businesses*, Irving Blackman, Probus Publishing Company, 1986, p. 75.

[xii] "Large Site Networks Quietly Take the Field," *CenterWatch*, August 2001, Vol. 8, Issue 8, Steve Zisson, p. 1.

[xiii] "A Bitter Pill for SMOs," *CenterWatch*, September 2000, Vol. 7, Issue 9, CenterWatch Editorial, p. 9.
[xiv] Ibid., p. 10.
[xv] Ibid., pp. 10-11.

CONCLUSION

If I've done the job I set out to do, you have gained many insights on how to grow your investigative site prudently and methodically by reading this book. You have also been able to determine from the criteria I have described whether you need to grow your site now or can wait a little while.

The guide should direct you in a step-by-step fashion to grow your site into a larger research center. Use the first half of the book about operating infrastructure to learn ways you can get your site ready to accept more studies. Expanding the size of the investigative site, both physically and in terms of capabilities, are important first stages of growth. This guide is written to prevent you from constantly playing catch-up when you attract more studies. It is also meant to help you understand how to identify and secure the number and types of studies you need in order to justify the size of your site, once you have grown it.

The second half of the book was written to help explain and give examples of the tools needed to improve operating controls and processes. What you might have been able to get away with as a smaller site will not work well as a larger one with more studies. This second half should give you some guidance on how you can become more organized at your investigative site and how you can prepare for upcoming regulations and technology.

The last chapter details how to devise an exit strategy for your investigative site. It explores the different conditions under which you might sell and helps you to value your site, independent of others' input.

The ultimate purpose of this book is to prepare the investigator as much as possible to grow his or her investigative site in a logical and manageable way by first evaluating if growth is desirable and feasible and then taking the proper steps toward achieving that growth in a controlled and organized way. But another important purpose is to make out of what is unknown and what may seem abstract a tangible plan of action. By reading my book, you've already taken that first important step.

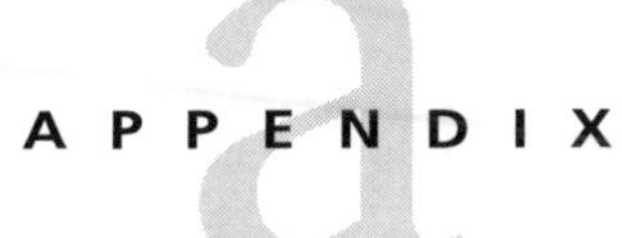

APPENDIX a

Growing the Site

Monitoring Visit Items

Monitoring Visit Items
Review of investigational drug supply and comparison to documentation
Review of regulatory study document file
Review of facilities and equipment
Verification of investigator compliance with protocol and any amendments
Verification that investigator and staff are adequately informed about the trial
Verification that the investigator has accurately prepared and provided all required reports to the sponsor, IRB, institution, and that each document is complete, accurate, dated, legible and properly identifies the trial
Notification of the investigator of any CRF discrepancy, entry error, omission or illegibility

Monitoring Visit Items (continued)

Monitoring Visit Items
Verification that the CRF corrections are made with dated, initialed documentation and explained, if required
Verification that essential documents are maintained
Communication of deviations from procedures, GCP or the protocol to the investigator, and the actions required to secure compliance
Training of the investigator and/or staff in areas that require additional training
Review of informed consent documents for each subject
Review of CRFs and comparison to source documentation (i.e., medical record)
Verification that only eligible subjects are enrolled
Verification that any therapy modifications are documented
Verification that any missed visits, tests or procedures are accurately documented on subject's CRF
Verification that all subject withdrawals or dropouts are reported and explained
Verification that only authorized persons have written on CRF
Assessment of the financial status of the study and requesting payment in accordance with the study contract
Preparation of a report of monitoring findings (preliminary during the visit and final after the visit)

Source: The RAN Institute, Inc., Ruth Ann Nylen, Ph.D., 2001.

Data Management

CRFs Received:

Date	#CRFs	Study #	Initials

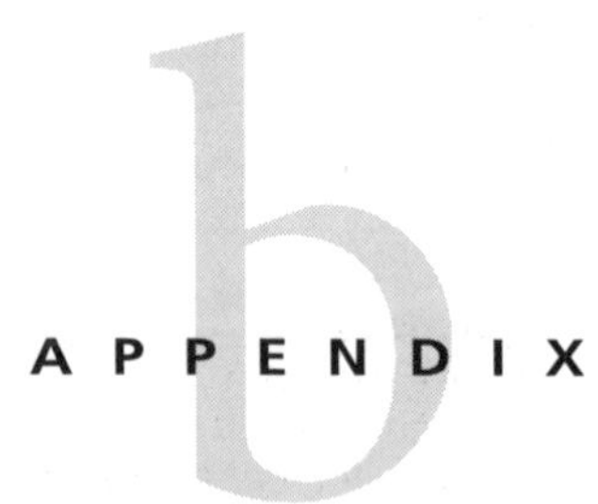

APPENDIX

Partnering with Investigators

Exhibit A

Investigator Agreement

This Agreement is made effective as of_________, by and between ________ Research, of_________, and _____________ M.D.

In this Agreement, the party who is contracting to receive services shall be referred to as _______Research, and the party who will be providing the services shall be referred to as _________M.D.

________M.D. has a background in the American Academy of Neurology and is willing to provide services to ___________Research based on this background.

_________Research desires to have services provided by _________M.D.

Therefore, the parties agree as follows:

1. DESCRIPTION OF SERVICES. Beginning on _________, ________M.D. will provide the following services (collectively, the "Services"):

> Sub-Investigator or Principal Investigator in Clinical Research Studies, all approved by _________M.D.
> Limited time to consult and offer opinions concerning possible studies.

2. PERFORMANCE OF SERVICES. The manner in which the Services are to be performed and the specific hours to be worked by Dr. shall be determined by Dr. _______Research will rely on Dr. to work as many hours as may be reasonably necessary to fulfill Dr. obligations under this Agreement.

3. PAYMENT. _________ will pay fees to _________ M.D. for the Services based on separate fee schedules for each contract. These fees shall be payable monthly, no later than the first day of the month following the period during which the Services were performed. Upon termination of this Agreement, payments under this paragraph shall cease; provided, however, that _________ M.D. shall be entitled to payments for periods or partial periods that occurred prior to the date of termination and for which Dr. has not yet been paid.

4. COMMISSION PAYMENTS. _________ will make commission payments to _________ M.D. based on gross 1.00% of payment for evaluable patients as per contracts. For the purposes of this Agreement, Contracts means Clinical Research Studies conducted by _________.

a. Accounting. _________ shall maintain records in sufficient detail for purposes of determining the amount of the commission. _________ shall provide to Dr. a written accounting that sets forth the manner in which the commission payment was calculated.

b. Death. If Dr. dies during the terms of this Agreement, Dr. shall be entitled to payments or partial commission payments for the period ending with the date of Dr. death.

5. SUPPORT SERVICES. _________ will provide the following support services for clinical research studies conducted by _________.

Dr.:
- Staff and secretarial support
- Clinical Research Coordinators
- Regulatory preparation
- File storage and maintenance

6. TERM/TERMINATION. This Agreement may be terminated by either party upon 90 days, written notice to the other party.

7. RELATIONSHIP OF PARTIES. It is understood by the parties that Dr. is an independent contractor with respect to _________ and not an employee of _________. _________ will not provide fringe benefits, including health insurance benefits, paid vacation, or any other employee benefit for the benefit of Dr.

8. DISCLOSURE. Dr. is required to disclose any outside activities or interests, including ownership or participation in the development of prior inventions, that conflict or may conflict with the best interests of _________. Prompt disclosure is required under this paragraph if the activity or interest is related, directly or indirectly, to:

- Any activity that Dr. may be involved with on behalf of _________
- Clinical Research

9. EMPLOYEES. Dr.'s employees, if any, who perform services for _________ under this Agreement shall also be bound by the provisions of this Agreement.

10. ASSIGNMENT. Dr.'s obligations under this Agreement may not be assigned or transferred to any other person, firm, or corporation without the prior written consent of _________.

11. CONFIDENTIALITY. Dr. recognizes that _________ has and will have the following information:

- machinery
- future plans
- trade secrets
- customer lists
- apparatus
- process information
- technical information
- business affairs

and other proprietary information (collectively, "Information") which are valuable, special and unique assets of _________. Dr. agrees that Dr. will not at any time or in any manner, either directly or indirectly, use any Information for Dr.'s own benefit, or divulge, disclose, or communicate in any manner any Information to any third party without the prior written consent of _________. Dr. will protect the Information and treat it as strictly confidential. A violation of this paragraph shall be a material violation of this Agreement.

12. UNAUTHORIZED DISCLOSURE OF INFORMATION. If it appears that Dr. has disclosed (or has threatened to disclose) Information in violation of this Agreement _________ shall be entitled to an injunction to restrain Dr. from disclosing, in whole or in part, such Information, or from providing any services to any party to whom such Information has been disclosed or may be. _________ shall not be prohibited by this provision from pursuing other remedies, including a claim for losses and damages.

13. CONFIDENTIALITY AFTER TERMINATION. The confidentiality provisions of this Agreement shall remain in full force and effect after the termination of this Agreement.

14. NON-COMPETE AGREEMENT. Recognizing that the various items of Information are special and unique assets of _________, Dr. agrees and covenants that for a period of 90 days following the termination of this Agreement, whether such termination is voluntary or involuntary. Dr. will not directly or indirectly engage in any business competitive with _________. This covenant shall apply to the geographical area that includes, but is not limited to, (I) engaging in a business as owner, partner, or agent, (ii) becoming an employee of any third party that is engaged in such business, or (iii) becoming interested directly or indirectly in any such business, or (iv) soliciting any customer of _________ for the benefit of a third party that is engaged in such business. Dr. agrees that this non-compete provision will not adversely affect the livelihood of Dr.

During the period of the Contractor's relationship with the Corporation, he shall not, directly or indirectly, alone or as a consultant to or as a partner, employee, officer, director, owner, or shareholder, be engaged in any activity that competes with the activities of the Corporation, or any of its subsidiaries or affiliates, without the prior written approval of the Corporation. Such approval may be granted or withheld in the sole discretion of the Corporation.

15. RETURN OF RECORDS. Upon termination of this Agreement, Dr. shall deliver all records, notes, data, memoranda, models, and equipment of any nature that are in Dr.'s possession or under Dr.'s control and that are _________'s property or relate to _________'s business.

16. NOTICES. All notices required or permitted under this Agreement shall be in writing and shall be deemed delivered when delivered in person or deposited in the United States mail, postage prepaid, addressed as follows:

If for _________:

_________ Research
Addressee
Street Address

If for Dr.:

_________ M.D.
Street Address

Such address may be changed from time to time by either party by providing written notice to the other in the manner as set forth above.

17. ENTIRE AGREEMENT. This Agreement contains the entire agreement of the parties and there are no other promises or conditions in any other agreement whether oral or written. This Agreement supersedes any prior written or oral agreements between the parties.

18. AMENDMENT. This Agreement may be modified or amended if the amendment is made in writing and is signed by both parties.

19. SEVERABILITY. If any provision of this Agreement shall be held to be invalid or unenforceable for any reason, the remaining provisions shall continue to be valid and enforceable. If a court finds that any provision of this Agreement is invalid or unenforceable, but that by limiting such provision it would become valid and enforceable, then such provision shall be deemed to be written, construed, and enforced as so limited.

20. WAIVER OF CONTRACTUAL RIGHT. The failure of either party to enforce any provision of this Agreement shall not be construed as a waiver or limitation of that party's right to subsequently enforce and compel strict compliance with every provision of this Agreement.

21. APPLICABLE LAW. This Agreement shall be governed by the laws of the State of _________.

Party receiving services:

_________ Research

By: ______________________________

Party providing services:

_________, M.D.

By: ______________________________

Exhibit B

Consultant Agreement

THIS AGREEMENT, made and entered into as of _________, by and between XYZ Center ("_________") and Doctor X, M.D. ("the Consultant").

WITNESSETH:

WHEREAS _________, a Site Management Organization and

WHEREAS the consultant has particular talents that may prove beneficial and useful to the Company, and

WHEREAS _________ wishes to enter into a Consulting Agreement on a per diem basis in connection with particular projects in relation to clinical research; and

WHEREAS the Consultant is willing to perform services for _________ upon the terms and conditions set forth in this Agreement;

NOW THEREFORE, in consideration of the premises and the mutual premises set forth hereafter, the parties agree as follows:

1. AGREEMENT TO PROVIDE SERVICES

_________ hereby agrees to use the Consultant to perform the services set forth in this Agreement for the Term of this Agreement, and the Consultant agrees to perform such services for _________ for the term of this Agreement, all upon the terms and conditions set forth hereafter.

2. SERVICES TO BE RENDERED BY THE CONSULTANT

_________ intends to utilize the services of the Consultant, including but not limited to his expertise in patient recruitment, clinical research experience, and as a liaison for professional and patient contacts.

3. TIMING OF SERVICES TO BE RENDERED

The Consultant agrees to make himself available to perform the aforesaid services at reasonable times. The parties agree that such services may be performed by the Consultant upon an agreed schedule set by _________ and the Consultant. It is further understood that substantial periods of time may pass during which no services are required of the Consultant, but such an occurrence shall in no way invalidate this Agreement or be deemed a breach of this Agreement by either party.

4. FEES & EXPENSES

_________ agrees to pay the Consultant at the various agreed upon rates for all services rendered.

5. **INDEPENDENT CONTRACTOR**

(a) It is understood and agreed by the parties that the Consultant is not an employee of _________. All rights, duties, and obligations of the parties, one to the other, are set forth in this Agreement and their relationship to each other is defined by the terms of this Agreement.

(b) No amounts paid to the Consultant by _________ pursuant to this Agreement shall be considered wages for the purpose of the Federal Insurance Contributions Act, the Federal Unemployment Tax Act, or the Collection of Income Tax at the Source of Wages Act.

(c) Since the Consultant's duties hereunder are not those of an employee, _________ shall make no attempt to control the manner in which the Consultant carries out the services to be performed hereunder.

6. **ASSIGNMENT**

_________ may not assign its rights under this Agreement without the prior written consent of the Consultant. The Consultant's duties hereunder are personal and may not be assigned without the prior written consent of the Consultant.

7. **TERM OF AGREEMENT**

The term of this Agreement shall be as long as both parties agree to continue the relationship. Notwithstanding the foregoing provisions, either party may terminate this Agreement upon thirty (30) days prior written notice to the other.

8. **MISCELLANEOUS**

(a) This Agreement shall be binding upon and shall insure to the benefit of the respective heirs, executors, administrators, successors, and assigns of the parties hereto.

(b) This Agreement may only be amended by an Agreement in writing executed by the parties hereto.

(c) This Agreement shall be governed by the laws of the State of _________.

IN WITNESS WHEREOF, the parties hereto have executed this Agreement as of the day and year above first written.

____

Consultant Signature Date

____

Site Signature Date

Exhibit C

Confidentiality Agreement

This Agreement, made this_________ day of _________ (month), ____ (year), by and between _________ , having its principal place of business at _________ (address).

Discussions have indicated that you have an interest in establishing an agreement with us concerning a potential relationship in regard to conducting clinical research trials.

In order for us to evaluate your potential site, it is necessary that we disclose certain Confidential Information relating thereto, stating that we have the right to disclose such Confidential Information to you for such purpose. It is also necessary that you disclose to us such Confidential Information relating thereto, stating that you have the right to disclose such Confidential Information to us for such purpose. We propose that the disclosure be made on the following basis:

As used herein "Confidential Information" shall mean any and all information, know-how and data, technical or non-technical, which relate to clinical research trials and which are disclosed in connection with the aforesaid discussions and evaluations.

In consideration of such disclosure, you agree not to use such Confidential Information for any purpose other than such evaluation, nor to disclose to any third party—unless otherwise agreed to in writing—any such Confidential Information or the fact that we have disclosed such Confidential Information to you and that you are making such evaluation at any time during this evaluation or thereafter for a period of 10 (ten) years, except as follows:

1. to the extent that such Confidential Information was known to you (from sources other than _________ or its affiliates) prior to its disclosure to you by or on our behalf and is documented in written record made by you prior to such disclosure; or

2. to the extent that such Confidential Information of fact is public knowledge prior to or after its disclosure, other than through acts or omissions attributable to you or your employees; or

3. to the extent that such Confidential Information was disclosed to you by a third party who did not derive such information from _________ or its affiliates.

You also agree to reveal such Confidential Information, and the fact thereof, only to those employees of yours and companies controlled by you who, in your judgment, have need to know such Confidential Information and the fact thereof.

You agree to make such evaluation as promptly as possible and upon our request return any or all Confidential Information together with all copies thereof, at any time but not later than 4 (four) months after receipt of the Confidential Information.

In turn, we agree not to use such Confidential Information for any purpose other than such evaluation, nor to disclose to any third party—unless otherwise agreed to in writing—any such Confidential Information or the fact that you have disclosed such Confidential Information to us and that we are making such evaluation at any time during this evaluation or thereafter for a period of 10 (ten) years.

We also agree to reveal such Confidential Information, and the fact thereto, only to those employees of ours who in our judgment, have need to know such Confidential Information and the fact thereto.

We agree to make such evaluation as promptly as possible and upon your request return any or all Confidential Information together with all copies thereof, at any time but not later than 4 (four) months after receipt of the Confidential Information.

If the foregoing is acceptable to you, please so indicate by signing this letter and returning it to us, whereupon it shall constitute a binding agreement between our companies.

Sincerely,

____

Signature Date

Accepted and agreed to:
Clinic name ______________________________

____

Signature of Representative Date

____

Printed Name Title

Exhibit D

Employment Agreement

This agreement is made this _________ day of _________ (month, year) by and between_________ (hereinafter referred to as "Employer") and _________ (hereinafter referred to as "Employee").

WITNESSETH:

In consideration of the employment by Employer of Employee, of the covenants and agreements of the parties hereto, respectively, as set forth hereinafter, and of other good and valuable consideration the receipt and sufficiency of which are hereby acknowledged, the parties hereto covenant and agree as follows:

1. The Employer hereby employs Employee and Employee hereby accepts employment under the terms and conditions hereinafter set forth.

2. The term of this agreement shall commence on and shall continue for one (1) year unless otherwise terminated as provided herein. If at the end of the initial term of the agreement the employee has fully and satisfactorily performed all of the obligations of the Employee, and Employee wishes to continue in the employment of Employer under the obligations and conditions of this Agreement, then the term of this Agreement shall renew automatically for successive one year terms and all of the obligations of the parties one to the other set forth in this Agreement shall continue in full force and shall be binding on the parties. Notwithstanding the foregoing provisions, Employee shall be entitled to terminate this Agreement for any reasons upon four (4) weeks written notice to Employer.

3. For all services rendered by Employee under this Agreement, Employer shall pay Employee an annual salary of $_________, payable in equal installments in accordance with Employer's normal payroll cycle, but in no event to be payable less frequently than every fourteen (14) days. In the event the term of this Agreement begins on a day other than the first day of the payroll cycle, the amount of the initial installment shall be prorated for such period.

4. Employee is engaged as a Study Coordinator to provide the supervision and management necessary to conduct on behalf of the Employer such clinical research trials as the Employer may designate from time to time, as well as such other services as Employer shall reasonably assign from time to time.

5. Employee shall devote full time, attention and energy to the business of the Employer and to the fulfillment of the Employee's functions as herein set forth.

6. Employee shall be entitled to ___ week(s) of vacation for each Employment Year during the term of the Agreement, during which time Employee's compensation shall be paid in full. After two years of service, employee shall be entitled to ___ weeks of vacation.

"Employment Year" as used herein means each twelve (12) month period for which the Employee is employed under the terms of the Agreement, the first Employment Year beginning on the commencement date stated in paragraph 2. Vacation shall be taken at such times as approved in advance by employer, such approval not to be unreasonably withheld. Employee shall also be entitled to such medical and dental benefits, retirement benefits, personal leave and other benefits, if any, as may be established from time to time by Employer for the benefit of its employees, subject to the qualification and eligibility requirements of the plan or plans establishing the benefits.

7. If employee dies during the term of this Agreement, Employer shall pay Employee's estate or personal representative the compensation to which Employee would be entitled for the week in which death occurred.

8. This Agreement may be terminated by Employer upon the occurrence of any of the following event.

(a) Death of employee;

(b) Disability of Employee which continues for more than sixty (60) days in any Employment Year. Employee shall be deemed to be "disabled" within the meaning of this Paragraph 8 if pursuant to an illness, accident or injury, the Employee is substantially unable to perform his/her duties as a full-time employee for a continuous period of sixty (60) days and within such sixty (60) day period the Employee's treating physician has rendered a medical opinion in writing to the effect that such disability is more likely than not to continue for more than ninety (90) days following the occurrence of such illness, accident or injury. The disabled Employee shall be deemed to be "disabled" as of the date of the illness, accident or injury.

(c) Employee's breach of any of the terms of the Agreement, including but not limited to failure to perform functions assigned to him/her thereunder in a proper and professional manner consistent with the industry standards;

(d) Conduct by Employee which causes public embarrassment or shame to Employee or which materially damages the business of the Employer;

(e) Any other conduct by Employee which Employer determines, in its sole discretion, to constitute good cause for Employee's dismissal.

(f) Lack of work opportunity within __________ to necessitate this position.

9. Employee recognizes and acknowledges that, in the course of his/her employment by the Employer, he/she may acquire information not generally known in the industry in which Employer is or may become engaged, which information Employer may desire to be and remain confidential (hereinafter referred to as "Confidential Information"). Employee recognizes and acknowledges that the wrongful use, misappropriations and/or disclosure of any such Confidential Information could constitute a breach of trust and could cause injury to the Employer, including, without limitation, damage to Employer's good will and competitive position. The Employee agrees to perform work as delineated within the contracts signed by Rx Trials, Inc. for the purpose of acquiring the clinical trial.

10. The Employee hereby agrees to hold and safeguard the Confidential Information in trust for the Employer, its successors and assigns, and agrees that he/she shall not, without the prior written consent of the Employer, misappropriate or disclose or make available to anyone for use outside the Employer's organization any of the Confidential Information at any time, during either his/her employment with the Employer or subsequent to the termination of his/her employment with the Employer for any reasons, including without limitation, termination by the Employer for cause or without cause.

11. Upon the termination of the Employee's employment with the Employer for any reasons, including without limitation, termination by the Employer for cause or without cause Employee shall:

(a) promptly deliver to the Employer all correspondence, drawings, manuals, letters, notes, notebooks, reports, flow charts, programs, proposals and any documents concerning the Employer's customers or concerning products or processes used by the Employer and, without limiting the foregoing, will promptly deliver to the Employer any and all other documents or materials containing or constituting Confidential Information.

(b) refrain from soliciting or inducing any employee of the Employer to leave the employ of the Employer and from hiring or attempting to hire any employee of the Employer, and

(c) not, directly or indirectly, own, manage, operate, join, control, or participate in the ownership, management, operation, or control of, or be connected in any manner with, any business within one hundred (100) miles of Employer's offices of the type and character of the business engaged in by the Employer for a period of eighteen (18) months from the date of the termination of the employment of the Employee.

(d) will not work in the area of clinical research for any physician/group/organization which has worked with _________ during the last 18 months for a period of 12 months following the termination of employee's employment.

12. The Employee acknowledges that a violation by the Employee of the provision of this Agreement could cause the Employer irreparable harm and damages resulting therefrom may be very difficult to ascertain. Accordingly, Employee covenants and agrees that in any event of a default in the provisions of this Agreement by the Employee, the Employer shall be entitled to specific performance of this Agreement, including but not limited to, injunctive and other equitable relief, in addition to all other remedies which may be available to the Employer under the law.

13. The covenants of the Employee set forth herein are the essence of this Agreement; they shall be construed as independent of any other provision in the Agreement.

14. The Employee hereby irrevocably submits to the jurisdiction of the United States District Court for _________ or the Circuit Court of _________ in any action or proceeding arising out of, or relating to, this Agreement; and the Employee hereby agrees that all claims in respect of any such action or proceeding may be heard and determined in either such court. The Employee agrees that a final judgment in any such action or proceed-

ing shall be, to the extent permitted by applicable law, conclusive and may be enforced in any other jurisdiction by suit on the judgment or on any other matters provided by applicable law related to the enforcement of judgment.

15. Wherever herein used the feminine gender shall include the masculine and neuter genders.

16. This Agreement shall be binding upon, and insure to the benefit of, the parties hereto, and the rights and obligations of the employer under this Agreement may be assigned by the Employer and shall insure to the benefit of and shall be binding upon its successors and assigns.

17. This Agreement shall be governed by the laws of the State of _________. The invalidity or unenforceability of any provision hereof shall in no way affect the validity or enforceability of any other provision.

18. The Employee acknowledges he/she has received and agrees to the duties, responsibilities, policies and procedures, and benefits provided or expected of him/her by the Employer.

IN WITNESS WHEREOF, the parties hereto have executed the Agreement as of the day and year first hereinabove written.

Employer

By: ______________________________

Employee

By: ______________________________

Exhibit E

Statement of Site Agreement

This Agreement is entered into by and between _________ (Your Name), a Site Management Organization with its principal office and place of business at __________________ (address), hereinafter called "_________ ," hereinafter called the "SITE" with a principal office and place of business at __________________.

1. **SCOPE OF WORK**

The SITE agrees to devote its best efforts to carry out the clinical research ("Research"), as set forth in the protocol, provided by _________ .

The SITE shall perform all the work under this Agreement as an independent contractor. The SITE is not an agent, employee, partner, representative or joint venturer of or with PBRC and nothing in this Agreement shall be construed to create such a relationship.

2. **PRINCIPAL INVESTIGATOR**

The SITE will identify the Principal Investigator who will be responsible for the direction of the Research at the SITE in accordance with applicable _________ and Sponsor policies which SITE warrants and represents are not inconsistent with the terms of this Agreement and the Protocol. If for any reason, the Principal Investigator is unwilling or unable to continue to serve as Principal Investigator and a successor, acceptable to _________ and the Sponsor is not available, this Agreement shall be terminated as provided in Article 14.

3. **PERFORMANCE PERIOD**

The SITE shall commence work upon receipt of the Materials from the Sponsor. Work shall be completed according to times specified in the attached Exhibit(s). This Agreement shall continue in effect unless terminated pursuant to the terms hereof, until the completion of the work described in the attached Exhibit(s) and upon payment of all fees and expenses to the SITE from _________ .

4. **RECORD KEEPING, REPORTING AND ACCESS**

A. It is agreed that the Sponsor or _________ authorized representative(s), and regulatory authorities to the extent required by law, may during regular business hours, arrange in advance with the SITE to:

(1) examine and inspect the SITE's facilities required for performance of the Research; and

(2) inspect and copy all data and work products relating to the Research.

B. The SITE shall perform the following record keeping and reporting obligations in a timely fashion:

(1) Preparation and maintenance of complete, accurately written records,

accounts, notes, reports and data of the Research. You agree to sign & date a statement in each patient's case report form attesting to your review and that the data are an accurate accounting of the treatment, care, and events surrounding the patient's involvement in the study. Federal regulations require that copies of case report forms be retained by the Principal Investigator for a period of no less than two years following either the approval the New Drug Application (NDA) or the withdrawal of the Investigational New Drug Application (INDA). To avoid any possible errors, you will contact the Sponsor prior to the destruction of any study records and will notify the Sponsor in the event of accidental loss or destruction of any study records.

Attention of the Principal Investigator is drawn to the fact that he may be subject to a field audit by inspectors of the U.S. Food and Drug Administration (FDA) or comparable foreign regulatory agencies and by representatives from _________ to verify that the study is conducted in accordance with the requirements of the Protocol, as well as in compliance with the federal regulations concerning the distribution and administration of Investigational New Drugs, and

(2) Preparation and submission to the Sponsor of all original case report forms ("CRFs") and electronic files (if applicable) for each patient or subject participating in the Research ("Research Subjects") as provided in the Protocol.

5. **COST AND PAYMENT**

A. As consideration for work performed under the terms of this Agreement, _________ agrees to pay the SITE as outlined on the attached Schedule A.

B. Payment shall be made payable to the SITE according to Schedule A appended hereto and incorporated herein by reference. All costs outlined on Schedule A shall remain firm for the duration of the Research, unless otherwise agreed to in writing by the SITE and _________ .

C. Reimbursements for any procedures, visits, or other charges performed apart from those scheduled by the protocol are the responsibility of the SITE.

6. **CONFIDENTIAL INFORMATION**

A. The SITE agrees not to disclose or to use for any purpose other than performance of the Research, any and all trade secrets, privileged records or other confidential or proprietary information (collectively "Information") disclosed to or developed by the SITE pursuant to this Agreement or any previous confidentiality agreement(s) relating to the Research. The obligation of non-disclosure and non-use shall not apply to the following:

(1) information at or after such time that it is or becomes publicly available through no fault of the SITE;

(2) information that is already independently known to the SITE as shown by its prior written records, provided that the SITE so advises the Sponsor promptly upon the SITE's discovery that the information is already independently known to the SITE;

(3) information at or after such time that is disclosed to the SITE on a non-confidential basis by a third party with the legal right to do so; or

(4) information required to be released by any governmental entity with jurisdiction, provided that the SITE notifies the Sponsor prior to making such release of information.

B. The obligations of the SITE under this Article shall survive and continue for five (5) years after termination of this Agreement.

C. The SITE shall hold in confidence the identity of the patient and shall comply with all applicable law(s) regarding the confidentiality of such records.

D. In the event the SITE finds it necessary to disclose information to a proper authority to permit the SITE to defend its research against an allegation of fraud, the SITE shall first notify __________ , and the SITE and __________ shall agree to a mutually satisfactory way to disclose such information as necessary for this limited purpose.

E. SITE agrees to hold the results of the study in confidence, subject to its rights under Article 7.

7. **PUBLICATION/PRESENTATIONS**

For any publication or presentation, a manuscript of the paper, abstract or other materials must be reviewed by the Sponsor prior to any outside submission. A period of fifteen (15) working days for presentation materials and abstracts and forty-five days for manuscripts will be required for the Sponsor's review. These requirements acknowledge the Sponsor's responsibility to evaluate such publications for their accuracy, to ascertain whether proprietary information (including trade secrets and patent protected materials) is being utilized and inappropriately released, to provide the investigator with information which may not yet have been available to him/her, and to provide input from co-authors regarding content and conclusions of the publication or presentation.

If an invention is described in a proposed publication which in the opinion of the Sponsor should be made the subject of a patent application, the SITE shall have four (4) months after full disclosure to the Sponsor to file such patent application. SITE shall withhold publication respecting that invention until such application is so filed by the Sponsor.

It is agreed that no presentation or publications will be authorized individually or by subgroups participating in the trial without the consent of all the relevant parties prior to publication of the pooled data, but in no event shall any SITE involved in this study be restricted from publishing independently after the expiration of twenty-four (24) months from the completion of Research.

8. **DATA, OTHER INFORMATION, INVENTIONS AND PATENTS**

A. All data, other information and inventions resulting from the performance of the Research shall be owned by the Sponsor and may be used and/or transferred by the Sponsor for any lawful purpose with no further payment to the SITE.

B. In the event that the Sponsor decides to file one or more United States and/or foreign patent applications covering one or more inventions resulting from the performance of the Research, the SITE and each Principal Investigator shall, at the Sponsor's request and expense, assist the Sponsor in the preparation and prosecution of such patent application(s) and shall execute all documents deemed necessary by the Sponsor for the filing thereof and/or for the vesting in the Sponsor of title thereto.

9. **PUBLICITY**

The SITE shall not use the Sponsor's name, nor issue any public statement about this Agreement, including its existence, without the prior written permission of _________ except as required by law (and, in such case, only with prior notice to the other party). The parties agree that in order for SITE to satisfy its reporting obligations, it may identify the Sponsor and _________ and the amount of funding received for the Research, but will not include in such report any information which identifies the name of the Research compound or the therapeutic areas of the Research.

10. **APPLICABLE LAW**

This Agreement shall be governed by the laws of the State of _________ .

11. **NOTICE**

Any notice required or permitted hereunder shall be in writing and shall be deemed given as of the date if it is (A) delivered by hand or (B) sent by registered or certified mail, postage prepaid, return receipt request, and addressed to the party to receive such notice at the address set forth below, or such other address as is subsequently specified in writing:

To _________:

For Contract/Payment Matters:
Name
Title
Site
Address

For Technical Matters:
Name
Title
Site
Address

For Administrative Matters:
Name
Title
Site
Address

12. **INDEMNIFICATION**

A. The Sponsor shall defend, indemnify and hold harmless the SITE (collectively the ("Indemnitees") from any and all liabilities, claims, actions or suits for personal injury or death directly arising out of or in connection with the administration or use of the drugs being studied through the Research ("Research Study Drugs") during the course of the Research; provided however:

(1) that the Research is conducted in accordance with the Protocol, all written instructions delivered by the Sponsor concerning administration of the Research Study Drugs or devices and Good Clinical Practice regulations,

(2) that such loss does not arise out of the negligence or willful malfeasance of any indemnitee, or any other person on the SITE's property, exclusive of _________ employees:

B. Deviations from the terms of the Protocol that may arise out of necessity do not constitute negligence or willful malfeasance and that SITE shall promptly notify _________ and the Sponsor in writing of any such deviations.

C. The SITE agrees that it will maintain during the performance of this Agreement the following insurance or self-insurance in amounts no less than that specified for each type:

(1) general liability insurance with combined limits of not less than $1,000,000 per occurrence and $1,000,000 per accident for bodily injury, including death, and property damage:

(2) Worker's Compensation Insurance in the amount required by the law of the state in which the SITE's workers are located and employer's liability insurance with limits of not less than $1,000,000 per occurrence; and

D. Upon request, the SITE will provide evidence of its insurance or self-insurance and, unless the SITE is self-insured, will provide to _________ thirty (30) days prior written notice of any cancellation in its coverage.

13. **SUBJECT INJURY**

The SITE shall contact the Sponsor for reimbursement for reasonable and necessary medical expenses incurred by Research Subjects for acute medical care, including hospitalization, in the treatment of adverse reactions arising directly from study drugs or devices following their administration or use in accordance with the Protocol, which expenses are not covered by the Research Subject's medical or hospital insurance coverage or other third party payor and are in no way attributable to the negligence or misconduct of any person in the employment of the SITE or to the Research Subject's own failure to follow instructions. No other compensation of any type will be provided by the Sponsor to the Research Subjects.

14. **TERMINATION**

A. This Agreement may be terminated by the SITE, _________ or the Sponsor for any safety and/or efficacy concerns, upon fifteen (15) days prior written notice.

B. In the event that the Sponsor or _________ exercises this right, reimbursement for costs and non-cancelable commitments incurred prior to the giving of such notice, will be limited to prorated fees based on actual work performed pursuant to the protocol. Any unexpended funds not due the SITE under this calculation but already paid to the SITE shall be returned to _________ within sixty (60) days of termination.

C. Immediately upon receipt of a notice of termination, the SITE shall stop entering Research Subjects into the Protocol and shall cease conducting procedures on Research Subjects already entered in the Protocol as directed by the Sponsor or _________, and to the extent medically permissible.

D. Termination of this Agreement by either party shall not affect the rights and obligation of the parties accrued prior to the effective date of the termination. The rights and duties under Articles 4, 6, 7, 8, 9, 10, 12, 13, 19, 20 and 21 survive the termination or expiration of this Agreement.

15. **ENTIRE AGREEMENT**

This Agreement represents the entire understanding of the parties with respect to the subject matter hereof. In the event of any inconsistency between this Agreement and the Protocol, the terms of this Agreement shall govern. The invalidity or unenforceability of any term or provision of this Agreement shall not affect the validity or enforceability of any other term or provision hereof.

16. **ASSIGNMENTS BY SITE**

This Agreement, and all rights and obligations hereunder may not be assigned by SITE without the express written consent of _________.

17. **CHANGES TO THE PROTOCOL**

Any alteration in or amendment to the attached Protocol or any additional clause in this Agreement must be approved in writing by the Principal Investigator, the IRB and the Sponsor prior to such alteration or amendment becoming effective. No financial adjustments shall be made because of such modification unless the parties hereto amend this Agreement accordingly.

18. **CONFORMANCE WITH LAWS AND ACCEPTED PRACTICE**

The SITE shall perform the Research in conformance with generally accepted standards of good clinical practice, with the Protocol, and with all applicable local, state, federal and foreign laws and regulations governing the performance of clinical investigations including but not limited to the Federal Food, Drug and Cosmetic Act and regulations of the FDA and comparable foreign agencies.

19. **DEBARMENT CERTIFICATION**

Neither the SITE nor any person employed thereby directly in the performance of the Research has been debarred under section 306(a) or (b) of the Federal Food, Drug and Cosmetic Act and no debarred person will in the future be employed by the SITE in connection with any work to be performed for or on behalf of _________ which may later become a part of any application for approval of a drug or biologic by the FDA. If at any time after execution of this contract, the SITE becomes aware that the SITE or any person employed thereby is, or is in the process of being debarred, the SITE hereby certifies that the SITE will so notify _________ and the Sponsor at once.

ACCEPTED AND AGREED:

FOR SITE:

____

Signature Date

____

Printed Name

____

Title

FOR __________:

____

Signature Date

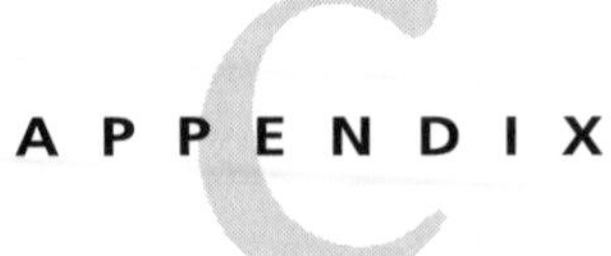

APPENDIX C

Improving Office Systems

Patient Data Form

Date: ____________________

Last Name: ____________________ First Name: ________________________

Address: ____

City: ______________________________ State: __________ Zip: ___________

Telephone: (Home) ___________ (Work) _____________ Fax: ____________

Occupation: ______________ Employer: _________ E-mail: _______________

List a number where you can be reached between 8:00 a.m.–5:00 p.m.

Age: _____ Date of Birth: _______ Sex: ______ Weight: ____ Height:______

Primary Physician: ____

Person to Contact in Case of Emergency: _____________________________

Address: ____

City: _______________________________ State: __________ Zip: __________

Telephone: (Home) ____________________ (Work) ______________________

Do you take any drugs regularly? (Circle) Yes No

Medication (Please list as many as possible):

____
____
____

Allergies (Please list as many as possible):____________________________

____
____

Do you smoke?	Yes	No
Do you drink alcoholic beverages?	Yes	No
Have you ever been hospitalized?	Yes	No
Have you ever had any kind of surgery?	Yes	No
Have you ever been told you are HIV positive?	Yes	No
AIDS?	Yes	No

IF YOU HAVE CALLED REGARDING STUDIES, PLEASE LIST WHICH ONES

____
____
____

SIGN-IN SHEET
CONFIDENTIALITY STATEMENT

By signing below I agree not to divulge the name of any patient or family participating in any program. Further, I agree to keep any and all treatment information concerning patients or their families in the strictest confidence.

Patient's name	Time	Patient's Name	Time
1.		21.	
2.		22.	
3.		23.	
4.		24.	
5.		25.	
6.		26.	
7.		27.	
8.		28.	
9.		29.	
10.		30.	
11.		31.	
12.		32.	
13.		33.	
14.		34.	
15.		35.	
16.		36.	
17.		37.	
18.		38.	
19.		39.	
20.		40.	

RECORDS RELEASE

To: ____

From: ____

Study: ____________________________ Coordinator: _________________

Documents requested: ________ Entire Chart (Do not send abstract)

________ Other _____________________________

Records Requested–From: __________________ To: ____________________

I hereby authorize you to release my medical records to:

Company Name
Address
Phone
Fax

Please Print Name: ____________________________ Date of Birth: _______

Social Security Number: _______-_______-_______

Signature: ____________________________ Date: _______________________

Witness: ______________________________ Date: _______________________

MEDICAL RECORDS TRACKING

Patient's Name	Date Requested	Study	Date Rec'd	Primary Coordinator

FORWARD INFORMATION TO PHYSICIAN FORM

___________ will notify your Primary Care Physician that you are participating in a Clinical Research study, *if you so choose*. Please note your decision below:

❍ Yes, Please notify my Primary Care Physician:

____

____

____

❍ No, Please DO NOT notify my Primary Care Physician.

____

Signature

DRUG DISPENSING LOG

Page _____ of _____

Sponsor: ______________________________ Protocol #: ________________________

Drug: ______________________________ * All shipping labels must be attached

Date	Pt. ID	Lot#	Bottle	Dispensed by:

DRUG TRANSFER LOG

Pharmaceutical Co.: ____________________ Study: ____________________

Date Transferred	To Facility	Amt.	By Whom	Date Returned	Amt. Returned

DRUG DISPOSITION LOG

Date: ______________________
Subject #: ___________________
Subject Int.: ________________

Date Dispensed	Amt. Dispensed	Date Returned	Amt. Returned	Counted by (init.)	Visit #

TELEPHONE LOG

Date: ______________________________ Time:_____________________

Conversation with: ______________________ Affiliation: ______________________

Telephone #: ____________________________ Fax #: ____________________________

Regarding: ____

_________ Placed Call _________ I Returned Call

_________ Party Called _________ Party Returned Call

____

____

____

____

____

____

____

____

____

____

____

Is action or follow-up necessary? ____ No ____ Yes (specify) ___________

____

____

____

Was action taken? ____ No ____ Yes (specify) __________________________

____

____

____

Signed: _________________________ cc: ________________________________

____

FREEZER

TEMP-CHEX™ TEMPERATURE RECORD

Date: ________ Temp. Range:____________ To:________ Year: _________

Month											
		Record	Initial	Record	Initial	Record	Initial	Record	Initial	Record	Initial
Day	1										
	2										
	3										
	4										
	5										
	6										
	7										
	8										
	9										
	10										
	11										
	12										
	13										
	14										
	15										
	16										
	17										
	18										
	19										
	20										
	21										
	22										
	23										
	24										
	25										
	26										
	27										
	28										
	29										
	30										
	31										

PATIENT RESPONSE CARD

Please take a moment to complete this card and place in the Patient Response Box. Your input will be helpful in maintaining and improving quality. Thank You.

Were you treated with respect during your entire visit?
❍ Yes ❍ No, what happened: ______________________________
____

Would you participate in a future study, if eligible?
❍ Yes ❍ No, why not: ______________________________
____

Has anything happened that you did **not** like?
❍ No ❍ Yes, what?: ______________________________
____

Has anything happened that you did like?
❍ No ❍ Yes, what?: ______________________________
____

Please use reverse for additional comments

TRACKING FORM FOR STUDY VISITS

*After screening and randomization visits, patients will return for visits 3, 4 and 5 between 1–3 days after their 72 hour Global Assessment in each cycle.

Pt. Name Phone#	Pt. ID#	Visit 1 Screening Day -10 to -1	2 Randomization Day 0	*3	*4	*5	Unscheduled

Coordinator(s): ______________________________

ADVERSE EVENTS

Protocol #: ____________________

Patient #: ____________________

Description	Start Date/ Time	Stop Date/ Time	Frequency 1 Single event 2 Intermittent 3 Continuous	Severity 1 Mild 2 Moderate 3 Severe	Study Drug Action Taken 1 None 2 Dose adjusted 3 Dose held 4 Discontinued	Med/TX Required 1 Yes Record CM 2 No	Drug Related? 1 Yes 2 No If no, specify etiology	Relationship to Device 1 Related please complete AE Device form 2 Unrelated	Serious? Yes/No	Outcome 1 cont'd Yes No 2 Resolved

IRB APPROVAL NOTICE

To: ____
____
____
____
____
____
____

Date: ___/___/___

Study: ____

Coordinator: ____

Please note that the above-referenced protocol has been approved and enrollment will begin soon. If you have not yet reviewed the protocol, please do so at your earliest convenience.

Should you have questions regarding study procedures, kindly contact the coordinator listed.

c: study coordinator